From Trauma to Harming Others

From Trauma to Harming Others shows the approach of professionals from the world-renowned Portman Clinic, which specializes in work with violence, delinquency and sexual acting out.

This book focuses on the intricacies of working with young people who display such worrying behaviours. Written by experienced and eminent authors, the chapters unpack central theories and open up original ideas describing a range of work with sexual offenders, compulsive pornography users and violent young people. The central theme of the book is trauma and how acting out can be understood as a way of managing the psychic pain of such trauma. The chapters are ingrained with understandings from the classical psychoanalytic traditions of the Portman and Tavistock Clinics, together with more recent thinking about trauma, rooted in neurobiological, developmentally and trauma informed theories. They emphasize the need for awareness of both the victim of trauma and the perpetrator within the same person presenting for help, while panning treatment.

With insights and examples from experienced clinicians, this book will be of value to all those working with traumatized, acting out young people.

Ariel Nathanson is a consultant child and adolescent psychotherapist. He is the clinical lead for the treatment of the under 21s at the Portman Clinic, where he has been working for many years, specializing in the assessment and treatment of children, adolescents and young adults who display perverse, delinquent and violent behaviours.

Graham Music (PhD) is consultant child and adolescent psychotherapist at the Tavistock and Portman Clinics and an adult psychotherapist in private practice. Formerly associate clinical director of the Tavistock's child and family department, he has managed a range of services working with the aftermath of child maltreatment and neglect and organized many community-based psychotherapy services.

Janine Sternberg is clinical course director of the IPCAPA (Independent Psychoanalytic Child and Adolescent Psychotherapy Association) training at the bpf. Previously, she worked as a Consultant Child Psychotherapist at the Portman Clinic, Tavistock and Portman NHS Trust, having worked for many years before that at the Tavistock Mulberry Bush Day Unit, a small unit for children with complex difficulties.

From Trauma to Harming Others

Therapeutic Work with Delinquent, Violent and Sexually Harmful Children and Young People

Edited by
Ariel Nathanson, Graham
Music, and Janine Sternberg

Routledge
Taylor & Francis Group

LONDON AND NEW YORK

First published 2022
by Routledge
2 Park Square, Milton Park, Abingdon, Oxon OX14 4RN

and by Routledge
605 Third Avenue, New York, NY 10158

Routledge is an imprint of the Taylor & Francis Group, an informa business

© 2022 selection and editorial matter, Ariel Nathanson, Graham Music and Janine Sternberg; individual chapters, the contributors

British Library Cataloguing-in-Publication Data
A catalogue record for this book is available from the British Library

Library of Congress Cataloging-in-Publication Data
A catalog record has been requested for this book

ISBN: 978-0-367-41554-9 (hbk)
ISBN: 978-0-367-41557-0 (hbk)
ISBN: 978-0-367-81521-9 (ebk)

Typeset in Times New Roman
by MPS Limited, Dehradun

Contents

Contributors

Anne Alvarez, PhD, M.A.C.P is a consultant child and adolescent psycho-therapist (and retired Co-Convener of the Autism Service, Child and Family Dep't. Tavistock Clinic, London, where she still teaches). She is author of Live Company: Psychotherapy with Autistic, Borderline, Deprived and Abused Children and has edited with Susan Reid, Autism and Personality: Findings from the Tavistock Autism Workshop. A book in her honour, edited by Judith Edwards, entitled Being Alive: Building on the Work of Anne Alvarez was published in 2002. She was Visiting Professor at the San Francisco Psychoanalytic Society in November 2005 and is an Honorary Member of the Psychoanalytic Centre of California. Her latest book, The Thinking Heart: Three Levels of Psychoanalytic Therapy with Disturbed Children was published in April 2012 by Routledge.

Patricia Allan is a child and adolescent psychotherapist at the Portman clinic, Tavistock and Portman NHS Trust and in private practice. She has a special interest in working with children who have suffered pre-verbal trauma, in understanding how this experience is stored in the body and the challenge for the therapist of finding non-verbal methods of working therapeutically with this type of trauma.

Dr Tim Baker is a child and adolescent psychotherapist at the Portman Clinic where he works with children, adolescents, young adults, groups and institutions. He also works for the Portman Forensic CAMHS team. Previously, Tim worked for a number of years at Simmons House adolescent in-patient unit and for the Anna Freud National Centre for Children and Families, for whom he continues to deliver trainings in 'Reflective Parenting' (Mentalization Based Treatment for parenting) and has also co-developed a group model of this intervention. Tim trained at the Tavistock Clinic and his doctoral research explored organizational dynamics in child and adolescent mental health teams.

Donald Campbell is a training and supervising analyst, distinguished fellow, past President of the British Psychoanalytical Society and former Secretary

General of the International Psychoanalytic Association. He also served as Chair of the Portman Clinic in London where he worked in outpatient psychoanalytic psychotherapy as a child, adolescent and adult analyst for 30 years with violent and delinquent individuals and patients suffering from a perversion. He has published papers and chapters on such subjects as adolescence, doubt, shame, metaphor, violence, perversion, child sexual abuse and horror film monsters. In 2017, his paper 'Self-analysis and the development of an interpretation' appeared in the *International Journal of Psychoanalysis.* Also, in 2017, he co-authored with Rob Hale, *Working in the Dark: Understanding the pre-suicide state of mind,* which was published by Routledge.

Ann Horne was a consultant child and adolescent psychotherapist at the Portman Clinic for almost 10 years. Trained in the classical and Independent traditions at the BAP (now IPCAPA at the BPF) where she became head of child psychotherapy training and of post-graduate development, she has written, published and taught in the UK and abroad, notably developing the independent psychoanalytic approaches with children and adolescents book series. Her selected papers – *On Children who Privilege the Body* – were published by Routledge in 2018. She is a fellow of the British Psychotherapy Foundation.

Graham Music (PhD) is consultant child and adolescent psychotherapist at the Tavistock and Portman Clinics and an adult psychotherapist in private practice. His publications include *Nurturing Children: From Trauma to Hope using neurobiology, psychoanalysis and attachment (2019), Nurturing Natures: Attachment and children's emotional, socio-cultural and brain development* (2016, 2010), *Affect and Emotion* (2001), and *The Good Life: Wellbeing and the new science of altruism, selfishness and immorality* (2014). He has a particular interest in exploring the interface between developmental findings and clinical work. Formerly associate clinical director of the Tavistock's child and family department, he has managed a range of services working with the aftermath of child maltreatment and neglect and organized many community-based psychotherapy services. He currently works clinically with forensic cases at The Portman Clinic. He teaches, lectures and supervises in Britain and abroad.

Ariel Nathanson is a consultant child and adolescent psychotherapist. He is the clinical lead for the treatment of the under 21s at the Portman Clinic, where he has been working for many years, specializing in the assessment and treatment of children, adolescents and young adults who display perverse, delinquent and violent behaviours. He has a private practice where he clinically works with adolescents and adults, and as an organizational consultant to residential communities and other frontline community-based care professionals.

Marianne Parsons is a child and adult psychoanalyst and a child and adolescent psychotherapist. Formerly head of clinical training at the Anna Freud Centre and Editor of the *Journal of Child Psychotherapy*, she worked with children and adolescents at the Portman Clinic from 1989 to 2008 where she developed a special interest in aggression and violence. She was a member of the Violence Research Group led by Mervin Glasser and ran the Portman Clinic Diploma in Forensic Psychotherapeutic Studies. Currently, she chairs the Training Analysis Committee for the Independent Psychoanalytic Child and Adolescent Psychotherapy Association and teaches and supervises widely on many psychoanalytic trainings.

Janine Sternberg is clinical course director of the IPCAPA (Independent Psychoanalytic Child and Adolescent Psychotherapy Association) training at the bpf. Previously, she worked as a Consultant Child Psychotherapist at the Portman Clinic, Tavistock and Portman NHS Trust, having worked for many years before that at the Tavistock Mulberry Bush Day Unit, a small unit for children with complex difficulties. She trained originally as a child psychotherapist at the Tavistock Clinic and subsequently as an adult psychotherapist at the BAP. She is more involved in training issues and active in the professional body for child psychotherapists, the ACP. She has been editor of the *Journal of Child Psychotherapy* and Editorial Co-ordinator of the BJP. In addition to numerous other chapters and briefer publications, she has written a book that addresses what capacities and skills are needed for psychotherapeutic work and how these may be enhanced by infant observation and co-edited (with Cathy Urwin) a book on infant observation as a research methodology.

John Woods was one of the staffs at the Portman Clinic for more than 20 years, working with both adults and young people. Originally an English teacher, he came to the Portman after experience in Special Education, Therapeutic Communities and Child and Adolescent Mental Health Service. Currently, a Member of the British Psychotherapy Foundation, the Institute of Group Analysis and the International Association for Forensic Psychotherapy, he is in private practice in London. Publications include *Boys Who Have Abused, psychoanalytic psychotherapy with victims/ perpetrators of sexual abuse,* Jessica Kingsley Publishers, 2003, co editor with Andrew Williams of *Forensic Group Psychotherapy,* Karnac 2014, `The Complaint` in Ryan, J (2007) ed *Remarkable Tales of Psychotherapy* Karnac, *Compromise; a play about Psychotherapy* Open Gate Press 2007, *Death of a Psychotherapist and Other Poems* Karnac 2017.

Introduction

Ariel Nathanson, Graham Music, and
Janine Sternberg

Trauma tears the fabric of which safety is made. When a sense of safety was established in childhood by a loving external and internal object, restoring this fabric is possible, potentially leaving a specific fragility or fault behind (Balint, 1979). At other times, when fear and abuse were chronic and relational, the fabric had to be specifically designed to sustain harm by avoiding pain, often by establishing control over external and internal objects that were either too intrusive or abandoning. Some of these fabrics, as will be described in this book, were tailor-made by a bad object, addictive in nature, exciting and harmful to self and others.

Although almost all our patients present to us with their various solutions to the relational traumas they endured, some appear to be still searching, disorganized, mentally and physically tossing and turning, never finding a right posture, even a pathological one, that actually works to reduce anxiety. This book will notice these patients too, maybe even as representing the chaotic stage in development from which all other patients found a way to extricate themselves.

Most of our other patients are not chaotic. They usually arrive in the aftermath of having done something harmful or following a crisis stemming from being caught up in an addictive destructive cycle that stopped working as a psychological solution. We work with young people presenting as sadistic, callous and unemotional, excited by their actions and feeling very little guilt or even shame. We see others, who might have harmed someone else, tormented with remorse and unable to integrate the way they perceive themselves with what they have done. Many of our patients enact their difficulties through the Internet, and quite a few chapters in this book relate to this theme. Pornography, at times very extreme images of sadomasochism, violence and child abuse, is quite a common enactment in our patient group, mainly adolescents and young adults. The use of the body in enactment and its connection to the mind is another focus in our clinical work. Some patients enact on their bodies, others break into other bodies and some might offer their bodies to be broken into, all devising different psychological solutions to similar relational traumas.

This book is about the way we make sense of these solutions relationally and how we work with the patients who present them.

Stephen King is a popular author of many horror books and thrillers, some of which have been made into popular films. His depiction of exciting horror and darkness is often similar to the way some of our patients are unable to enjoy life's activities without transforming them into exciting, dark, risk seeking endeavours, as if endlessly caught up in one of his narratives.

Nevertheless, King's (2011) personal introduction to William Golding's (1954) *Lord of the Flies* centenary edition is very interesting and in some way helps to link this classic tale to the subject of this book. In his introduction, King quotes the author reminiscing about telling his wife one day, 'wouldn't it be good to write a story about some boys…showing how they would really behave?' King focuses his introduction on his experience of reading the book for the first time aged 12, and the sense that the words 'reached out and grabbed him by the throat', as they corresponded to his actual experience of growing up. He says that the book was 'a perfect understanding of the sort of beings my friends and I were at 12 or 13, untouched by the usual soft soap and deodorant. Could we be good? Yes. Could we be kind? Yes again. Could we, at the turn of a moment, become little monsters? Indeed, we could. And did. At least twice a day and far more frequently on summer vacations, when we were often left to our own devices'.

Lord of the Flies directly correspond to the real emotional experiences of children and teenagers. It is compelling because of that, describing experiences as they are, rather than dividing those along the usual lines of 'good and bad' in order to market them in a way that makes them palatable, easy to identify with or reject.

Ralph is the book character favoured by many teenagers reading Lord of the Flies. It is easy to identify with his wish to protect and be a benevolent leader, rejecting Jack, the callous hunter who promoted fear and offered excitement and cruelty as protection from it. However, Golding did not make the teenage reader's life easy by making their experiences totally separate. Instead, in one powerful scene, Ralph joins Jack and the gang of children in murdering Simon, making the Ralph character experience the thrill of cruelty and joining in with the mob, creating inner conflict, confusion, psychic pain and difficulty stemming from the knowledge that what is done can never be undone.

As Child and Adolescents psychotherapists at the Portman Clinic know, it is impossible to separate the world into victims and perpetrators. Attempting to do so is similar to keeping Ralph away from the dark excitement in his own self. Yet, the social myth that bad people can and should be separated from good people and even banished is powerfully unavoidable even in those who consciously attempt to integrate.

A 19-year-old patient, who had been sexually abused by his older brother, was only able to disclose his own past abuse after being arrested for watching images of child abuse on the Internet. A few years into his treatment, he told his psychotherapist, 'I wish I was just a victim who could hate his abuser. I do hate him but what I hate more is that I understand him…that in my mind I can be him'. This patient longed to be 'just a victim', as he put it. As a victim he had a story that he felt he could tell. However, each time he felt the comfort of the victim position, dividing the world and seeing his own darkness only in others, his mind was interrupted by the intrusive knowledge of his own actions. This patient was severely traumatized by the abuse he suffered. At the time, the only solution to avoid the pain of being passively assaulted was to master it by divorcing his mind from his body. Whilst the mind shouted 'no', the body experienced some strange excitement and a sense of participation, which was then harnessed as a solution to psychological pain.

Relational abuse, such as just described, is not an abrupt assault that starts, damages and ends. It includes periods of grooming – a gradual sense of growing into an abusive relationship, or a dependency on an abuser and the relationship to them. In those situations, the capacity to say no or even understand what is going on, not to mention the concept of asking for help and stopping being hurt, slowly diminish or do not exist. The threat of losing the abuser by destroying them or the fear of being caught participating, feeling guilty and ashamed, all prevent access to a reality where being protected and feeling safe are readily available. As we know from our clinical experience, many people who groom and sexually harm others often say that the victim never said no. In parallel, many victims of relational abuse do not remember ever saying yes. Their experience is of a passive tolerance, a kind of a vague 'OK', which they might have even said as things gradually deteriorated.

As it is extremely difficult to survive a sense of constant passive suffering, the mind looks for other solutions to master trauma and regain a sense of active control. The patient described above, similar to many others, regained a sense of agency through enhancing the giddy, painful and sexual excitement he experienced in his body. The part of the mind supporting this participation and mastery, now operating in parallel to the passive suffering victim, started to creatively invent new ways of joining in, such as looking for sexualized images of children, normalizing the experience and taking action. Gaining mastery over relational trauma by enactment usually involves both the mind and the body. The solutions we encounter in our patients are always real actions, never only thoughts, feelings and fantasies. As such, they have an impact in the real world and consequences.

Ordinary life is full of chances to feel overpowered, humiliated or victimized within relationships, groups and organizations. Our young patients have parents and carers, go to school, live in residential units and go to work or university. They experience various types of sexual and non-sexual relationships, contact with authority, rules and boundaries. What we see and hear about when they present to us is how their old solutions continue to operate as they struggle to tolerate and cope with experiences which for example require tolerating emotional pain or using benign aggression. Unable to use their aggression assertively and constructively, fight for their rights in a self-protective constructive and appropriate way, they use their familiar old solutions and avoid extreme emotional experiences through action that often greatly disturbs others.

We do not only work with the Ralphs (Lord of the Flies, Golding, 1954), who might painfully mourn their lost innocence, attempting to integrate conflicting aspects of their developing personality. We also work with the Jacks, heavily reliant on risk taking, survival through adopting a gang state of mind (Rosenfeld, 1971), and excitement, and even with the Rogers, who Alvarez writes about in her chapter – callous and cold, excited by the harm they inflict on others. With them, and others described in this book, it is a mistake and often a trap to address the victim in the patient and turn a blind eye to the callous perpetrator who hides his excitement or even sniggers in contempt.

Not all patients are callous and sadistic, but enactment is almost always the reason for them being seen at the Portman. 'What has he done?' is the usual first question in our intake meeting, and relationally understanding the action is our first task in assessing a patient for psychotherapy. From the beginning, our attitude and technique are quite different to the usual. We would not accept referrals of patients who only suffer with disturbing and painful thoughts, feelings or fantasies or who present solely as victims of trauma. In our assessment, we make sure that our future patients do not deny their actions and are able to take responsibility for those or at least acknowledge them. With young patients we make sure that they are held and understood by a network of professionals and carers, who clearly recognize the issues at hand and do not deny risk, even if the young person is too disturbed to communicate and relate clearly.

A 15-year-old boy was referred by the youth offending service after being convicted for the sexual abuse of his half sister. Now in care, rejected by his family, he presented as suicidal and mortified by what he had done. His assessing psychotherapist felt as though the mild mannered suffering young man talking to her in the consulting room could not have been the same boy who raped his sister. Indeed, like many similar cases he was a very 'good boy' who would never get angry and aggressive. Compliant, he always wanted to do well and never be like his own father who was controlling and violent to his mother and left when the patient was younger. He described the abuse as something that happened gradually, always expecting his sister to tell him to stop or tell their mother, constantly promising to himself that he would stop but later finding himself doing it again and escalating. Like most of our other patients, this young man was unable to articulate any thought or feeling relating to what he did whilst he was still engaged in action. Thought and the verbal communication of feelings and emotions is totally replaced by action and excitement. At the time of his enactment, this patient was still a very compliant young man, never angry, unaware of his intense envy, aggression and sense of being rejected by his mother who preferred his sister to him.

What makes young people turn to action that hurts others rather than developing other, even pathological, solutions? Perversion, 'the sexual form of hatred' as defined by Stoller (1975), is fundamental to the way psychotherapists at the Portman understand the actions of their patients. However, although the 15-year-old patient described above had definitely taken a perverse solution to his difficulties, he is different to an adult Portman patient who had been doing so habitually over many years, totally dependent on this addictive cycle, which had yielded further real damage and consequences.

Indeed, although almost all habitual sex offenders started enacting in adolescence or even before, only a minority of adolescents who sexually harm others turn into habitual sex offenders. The reason for this, in our clinical experience, is that the actions of young people are actually quite diverse and in the context of their adolescent development. Although the action might look the same, its meaning is varied and depends on the relational environment that produces it. The 15-year-old patient described here, for example, was not sexually attracted to children. His attack was an expression of hatred, aimed at hurting his mother's special child.

Similarly, violent and delinquent young people are different to the seasoned, often antisocial personality disordered patient seen as an adult. We define violence, following Glasser (1979), as hurting someone else's body, rather than having violent feelings and fantasies. In addition, still following Glasser (1979), we differentiate between self-preservative violence in the context of fighting for survival, and sadistic violence, self-gratifying, addictive and designed to control the object. Many of our highly traumatized and disorganized young patients are violent. These types of patients are familiar to many readers of this book who are not psychotherapists – care workers, social workers, teachers and assistants. They are the ones who attack their therapists in their sessions and challenge individuals and organizations in their struggle to contain them. Most of them, as will be described later in this book, especially by Patricia Allan, were not even able to organize around a specific enactment to serve as a solution to their traumatic experiences. Although they might not be strangers to perverse excitements and sadistic violence, they are mostly reactive and disorganized. Others are violent and criminal within the organization of a gang, which also provides them with purpose, belonging, safety, money and sex, as an antidote to a daily life of fear and trauma. Only a minority of violent young people will become the violent adults that attend the Portman, broken down, after years in prison, paranoid and impulsive.

At this point in time, Portman young patients grew up and live within a social and technological environment that adult patients (and indeed most psychotherapists) never encountered as children. Their use of the Internet, social media and pornography is unprecedented and not always easy to understand and decipher from what should be expected as the current norm. Some patients, for example, would talk about finding their father's collection of pornographic magazines, as they began to look for similar thrills online. Those talking about their experience at the end of the 1990s and the beginning of the 2000s, would talk about slow modems, discussion groups, exchanging images with others or needing to pay and not having a credit card. Those describing the same excited quest after 2007, when free pornography became ubiquitous and organized by complicated algorithms, will describe never ending and escalating session of clicking images and videos, unable to tear themselves away. Others, even later, will talk about the dark net, being invisible and attempting to find dark, sadistic and violent images, or delinquently and criminally buying drugs or weapons to sell and use.

How to help those who hurt and disturb others? Many would rather not to attend to this question at all and leave it to others. Some would say that it is completely inappropriate to help those who have hurt, seeing help as collusion and denial rather than an appropriate consequence to harmful actions. The British Home Secretary, Priti Patel, was quoted when relatively new saying that her office would make people safer by '...putting the fear back into criminals and perpetrators'. However, we see that traumatized victims/perpetrators are experts in avoiding fear and other feeling states by swiftly translating those into action. 'Putting the fear back' is what they do best and turning this into government policy can only result in an endless cycle of escalation. Many of our victim/perpetrator patients would join the politician's sentiments as they endlessly ruminate about taking revenge against those who hurt them, only to later feel overwhelmed and defeated, experiences they need to eradicate through harm – putting the fear and humiliation into someone else.

Yet, it would be a mistake to see the Home Secretary's statement as only representing a populist reactive agenda. It also relates to the real experience of those working with young people who are violent and extremely disturbing. The wish to punish and put the fear back into the young person who produced it is familiar and natural. Similarly familiar is the opposite response of trying to excuse harmful behaviour, address people only as victims, placate and dismiss, as a way of avoiding the disturbing impact the work has on those who dare to get close (Drysdale, 1968). Obviously, both being punitive and adopting a placatory position does not make these enacting patients feel safe and would therefore only escalate their behaviour and disturbed states of mind. Being overpowered in a humiliating way will enflame their need for taking revenge, and being placatory will increase their sense of control and sadism.

The therapeutic position that this book is focused on making can only be available by recognizing the pull into the other two options described here. Being conscious of one's own experience helps in adopting this third option, at times an elusive therapeutic stance, hiding in the valley between collusion and punishment, beyond sadism and masochism. Finding this position is a not a simple technical challenge. In fact, at times it constitutes the main part of the work, especially in the work with psychopathic young people. In psychotherapy, we attempt to take a non-judgemental position in which we offer our patients the opportunity to think safely about their actions, understand those, notice their impact on themselves and others and slowly translate them back into the form the enactment attempted to avoid. Almost all the authors in this book address this challenge conceptually and technically, trying to answer the question of 'how do we treat these patients'.

Child and Adolescent psychotherapists are trained to work with patients who act in and outside sessions. Children play and move, challenging their therapists to make sense of their behaviour and find symbolism in played-out narratives. Adolescents act out, defy authority and experiment, expecting their therapists to respond. Many patients in psychotherapy describe their experiences with much pain and suffering and most Portman patients are no different. However, if we only listen to the narrating patient in the room, suffering the emotional and practical consequences of the enacting patient outside the room, we would soon be colluding with the victim whilst neglecting, fearing and placating the perpetrator, re-enacting the patient's personality structure and life experience.

Here lies one of the biggest difference between regular psychotherapy and Portman work – the therapeutic focus on both victim and perpetrator and the fundamental need to fully understand the perpetrator's actions; the addictive excitement, the sadism and masochism, the control and mastery, and the idea that there is very little that could compete with these solutions in avoiding extreme and unbearable experiences such as engulfment, abandonment, fear, humiliation, envy and hatred.

As a young patient who used to be violent to his girlfriend once said, 'it is only after I stopped being violent to her that I started feeling terrified that she might leave me'. Those not understanding the nature of sadomasochistic relationships might be perplexed by this comment – obviously, as long as he was hurting her he should have felt anxious that she would leave, not after he managed to stop. However, from our experience, as will be described in this book from a variety of angles, sadistic control is employed to avoid the anxiety of either being left or overwhelmed and engulfed (Glasser, 1979). Once control is abandoned, the anxiety and trauma at its base are experienced, at times in the most overwhelming way.

As reflected in the title of this book, chapters will look at trauma and taking action as a psychological solution to it. Our task as editors has been to collect the papers that best describe the way we think, understand trauma and relate to the meaning of enactment. Equally, as suggested in this introduction, providing help to those who harm others challenges both social norms and therapeutic practice. Chapters in this book will address this central aspect of our work and how our therapeutic technique developed to address these challenges.

The book opens with a chapter from Marianne Parsons that introduces the reader to concepts much used by Portman staff, such as the core complex, and the importance of recognizing the victim & the perpetrator within the same patient. It also highlights some ideas about how best to work with such young people and the importance of meticulous history taking. For readers unfamiliar with the concepts underlying the approach used by Portman clinicians this is a most useful starting point.

We move from there to chapters where the emphasis is on understanding the landscape that Portman patients inhabit and an attempt to think about how they may have come to be there. Using an updated version of a previously published paper, Anne Alvarez introduces us to the destructiveness of the psychopathic child, through both theory and brief clinical examples, and considers technical issues and 'the need to meet the psychopathic patient where he really is, in the inner bleak emotional cemetery'. She looks in minute detail at this world that many of us may prefer to avoid thinking about in order to 'distinguish between the kind of destructiveness which is motivated by anger, that by bitter hatred, that by outrage, that by sadism, and that by casual brutality'. She gives brilliantly vivid examples of work with patients, detailing where she has made mistakes and sharing what she has learned from those painful experiences. The chapter also, most helpfully, looks at what might be said, how and when, the need for coolness and 'minimalistic doses' to make contact with such patients. However, it also usefully recognizes situations where nothing might 'get through', helping to puncture grandiose rescue fantasies, which in themselves refute the depth of the patient's horrific inner experience. Yet at the same time she also encourages us to be alert to the tiniest 'flicker' that may denote something more hopeful. Alvarez is the only contributor to this book who has not worked directly at the Portman, but she has mentored and supervised many of us who have worked there and we are privileged to have her contribution to this book.

The following chapter by Don Campbell, a version of which has appeared before in a book of introductory essays on psychoanalysis, places thoughts about perversion centrally in its historical context. He starts with quotations from Freud that display Freud's own non-judgemental approach and understanding that 'the ego's task is to negotiate compromise where there is conflict between the inside and outside in order to achieve stability and balance'. Seen through this lens the development of a perversion is an attempt to resolve a problem, an attempt that may indeed be maladaptive, but may feel to the patient the only solution available. His chapter contains a masterly exposition of a concept much used at the Portman, the differentiation between self-preservative aggression and sadism, and he shows the ordinary development of sadism as the child's attempted solution to manage the 'ruthless' aggression he feels towards his mother. He carefully traces how the 'development from ruthless aggression to the libidinisation of aggression progresses to the intensification of sadism....(leading to) the development of perverse solutions to neurotic or psychotic conflicts'. Campbell also looks at aggression and considers briefly whether there is evidence for the death drive. The chapter includes a description of work with a young man who had sadistic fantasies about sex with young girls. As well as giving us a vivid picture of this young man, his various defences and attempted solutions, Campbell also looks at technique and the need to avoid collusion or an authoritarian approach, being aware of how much of the patient is indeed hidden not only from the therapist but also from the patient's conscious self.

Graham Music and Heather Wood's chapter on internet sex and pornography splendidly manages the difficult task of simultaneously taking a wide sweep, placing the problem in its social context, holding fast to its psychoanalytic perspective and being aware of the biological aspects of addiction. The problems that adolescents have to manage when forging a sexual identity, and how internet use may seem to aid, but in fact interfere with this, are addressed, with the idea that the screen can sometimes operate as 'an electronic transitional object'. We see Wood's vast experience and deep scholarship about the potentially damaging use of the internet (a theme repeated in John Woods' chapter) and together with Music she has produced a chapter that is likely to become a much valued resource for those wanting to look at these issues in a clear and balanced way. There are a number of case examples, the first of which helps us to understand what in the boy's background led him to use such defences. We are shown the work that was done by Music to help put him more in touch with the reality of his own body reactions. As with so many of the chapters in this book, we see adaptations to technique (here Music bringing in some techniques from Mindfulness) linking body states with states of mind, leading to the patient being able to become more in touch with himself. Other case examples follow, including one of a girl displaying herself online, where the despair and wish to be 'seen' are highlighted, and one of a young man whose interests were paedophilic.

John Woods' chapter also looks at internet pornography. He starts with a hard hitting exposition of the many problems that are exacerbated, if not caused, by the use of internet pornography, citing reports that show the impact that such use can have on adolescents: 'The child goes into adolescence assuming, for example, that women always want sex and that sex is nothing to do with relationships'. He contrasts this with ideas from Winnicott about the growth of relationships, the 'creating' of the other. He also links his concerns with other Winnicottian concepts, pointing out that there 'is a break between the subject and the viewed object. The object viewed over the internet usually cannot see the subject', unlike the importance of the mutual reciprocity of gaze between mother and baby of which Winnicott writes. The chapter considers how 'normal' use of internet pornography on occasions becomes compulsive and excessive, and examines the reasons for this. Using a relatively brief clinical example, Woods shows how the adolescent felt he was becoming 'invaded' by the violent imagery he accessed, withdrawing more from school and the outside world. Woods carefully traces his tentative involvement with another person, and the usefulness of no longer being in a 'no limits' world that the Internet had previously provided. His chapter helpfully suggests that it is possible for an adolescent to move away from reliance on Internet pornography if able to engage in therapy, perhaps especially if able to make use of a benign adult male.

When reading Ariel Nathanson's chapter, 'Mental hacking and back-room thinking', we are still within the world of the internet, but looked at from a different perspective, and also using the concept of hacking in both a real and a metaphorical way. His model of the 'backroom' ('The backroom functions as both a hiding place and a control centre') way of operating is one that so many of his colleagues have found invaluable. Through a lively and engaging brief description of his work with Andy, we get to understand both the specific ways of behaving and the traumas that they were designed to master or protect against; in Andy's case and others mentioned, a sense of intimacy and closeness. The chapter interestingly delineates various types of backroom presentations, giving brief examples to help the reader understand the distinctions he is making. The 'mental hacker' uses knowledge deliberately accumulated through manipulation as a way of feeling that he can exercise 'control of his victim, and denigrate and dismiss the need for care and attachment'. The emphasis on 'undercover' action, secrecy and deception permeate this paper. The 'backroom operator's usual sense of superiority, lack of concern for the other or guilt are shown to be valorized, treated as attributes which make engagement in therapy difficult. In a fascinatingly subtle way Nathanson looks at the avoidance of being discovered, which can leave the backroom operator feeling empty and unnoticed, flat despite all the efforts to generate excitement. He notes the risk of enactment from both therapist and patient in the consulting room and makes some suggestions about how therapists can be aware of, and incorporate lessons from the concept of the backroom into their interactions with some patients.

Graham Music's chapter, adapted from a previously published version, starts by starkly reminding us of the dreadful damage that some patients may have already inflicted on others. Again we see the view, central to this book, that the actions that have led the patient to come to the Portman are designed (unconsciously) to 'avoid the pain of core complex anxieties by maintaining a form of manageable contact with the object'. His chapter gives a very helpful understanding of Core Complex issues, and how 'a fear of being engulfed, leads to a sense of dread and aloneness which then becomes unbearable and in turn leads to clinging to the object, or in many patients, a need to take control and possession of it, often violently'. Music's differentiation between 'hot' and 'cold', also referred to, using different terminology, in other chapters within the book (e.g. Alvarez), can also usefully orientate clinicians as they struggle to understand what their patient is evoking in them. Music's special contribution to the field of child psychotherapy has been his interest in linking developmental research with psychoanalytic concepts, and this chapter also most usefully emphasizes the neurobiological factors, the physiological arousal that occurs in certain situations for patients who have previously suffered trauma and abuse. His work encourages all of us to be aware of the 'embodied countertransference' and make use of it in our work. We also see how his understanding, so firmly rooted in a familiarity with brain and biology, inevitably leads him to alter his technique. The descriptions of his empathic, rather 'vague' responses to Shane give us an insight into helpful ways of working with highly reactive children, while we see a more direct, challenging, approach to 'callous' Mick. The chapter also addresses the problems posed particularly by sexual aggression, with its additionally addictive quality.

We go from this to Ann Horne's chapter on 'Oedipal aspirations and phallic fears', a longer version of which has been previously published. Again we have the privilege to see a skilled clinician at work as she introduces us to Stanley, putting his perverse behaviour into context as an attempted solution to trauma, telling us that his particular circumstances 'left him with only the desperate manoeuvre of adopting a perverse solution'. She understands his fetishistic behaviour using both a developmental and a psychoanalytic frame-work. The chapter provides a scholarly, yet accessible, introduction to fetis-hism, concentrating on the more limited accounts within the psychoanalytic literature of it when shown by children. Horne's close detailed descriptions of her interactions with Stanley, letting us know what thoughts and feelings his behaviour evoked in her, show us an experienced, sensitive therapist working skillfully. She alerts us early on in the paper to her 'mistake' in arranging to see this 19 year old's parents without him, as if he were a much younger child, and on reflection thinks about the 'strong counter-transference pressure not to see Stanley as a potent male – and to recognise behind this his anxieties about being phallic and being perceived to be so'. All through Horne's descriptions of her work we get a great sense of her gentle humour, her accepting curiosity and her thinking mind, and there is acknowledgement of the setbacks which were accepted as a necessary part of the progress-another aspect of technical considerations that Portman clinicians are used to keeping in mind.

Tim Baker's chapter focuses on a comparison between male abusers and female self-harming patients who he had worked with in his previous setting, a residential unit. In doing this he is drawing attention to an idea much used by Portman clinicians, that of the 'victim within the perpetrator and vice versa'. The attack on parents and on self by becoming a 'sex offender' is noted. For some patients anxiety about separation, which is one of the tasks of adolescence, is seen as complicated and Baker hypothesizes that 'such perverse risk taking thus allows these adolescents to satisfy the development push to feel separate from their parents or parental figures whilst paradoxically keeping these adolescents ever more enmeshed with them'. As other authors in this book (e.g. Music and Wood) also do, he creates a composite to protect confidentiality, but ensures that he catches the essence of the dilemmas such patients feel and express. The patients he describes mask their aggression and hostility: in a wonderfully vivid way we hear of instances where a 'patient's aggression is expressed through victimhood and complaint, and ... the nature of its expression forecloses any straightforward response'. Baker notes how such a response also impacts on the therapist, stirring up a wish to confront the patient, Pietr, harshly with the reality of his sexually abusive act, noting that the patient was 'inviting me to victimise him with the truth so that instead of being in touch with being a perpetrator he could settle again into the familiar emotional state of misunderstood victim'. Baker sensitively considers the repetition within the therapy of the difficulties that he and his patients had in using aggression in a benign and straightforward way. The chapter links the vivid case material with useful theoretical ideas about over-intrusive, yet non-attentive, mothering and a sophisticated adaptation of Glasser's Core Complex to think about the difficulties of working with issues of intimacy without an early experience of being truly seen.

Patricia Allan's chapter shows us the determination often displayed by Portman clinicians when she writes about her work with younger, severely traumatized, disorganized children who do not respond to any form of verbal interpretation. As we have already noted, all the chapters give opportunity for thinking about ways of reaching and, if possible, helping deeply troubled patients. As we saw earlier in the chapter by Music and Wood, Allan attempts to make contact with Sean by deviating from 'standard technique'. Noting that he used his body as his main form of communication, over time, she too used her body (striding round the room in a way that mirrored Sean's actions) to show her understanding, not verbally specified, of his states. Allan gives wonderfully detailed descriptions of Sean's ways of being in the room with her, including honestly attending to her own reactions, 'wary and repulsed', to think deeply about his experiences. She introduces us to the many ways in which Sean presented himself-compliant, 'stupid' and 'perverse', and notes carefully when Sean used each, using her understanding to make sense of his responses: 'rather than attack me, Sean eroticised the aggression and invited me to join him in a perverse sexual coupling'. The chapter, which describes work with a child rather than an adolescent, also gives a wonderful insight into the way therapy can be useful, taking a playful approach, yet not abandoning the knowledge held by both therapist and patient that the task of therapy is an extremely serious one. Her paper also emphasizes the need for work with the network: using the strong image of shoring up the earthquake damaged building before entering it in an attempt to rescue the child, she delineates all the stages that a referral at the Portman needs to go through, before embarking on individual psychotherapy could be suggested, in order to ensure that the therapy does not destabilize the child and cause an already fragile system to break down.

The last clinically based chapter in the book is Ariel Nathanson's 'Embracing darkness: Clinical work with adolescents and young adults addicted to sexual enactments', a paper which was previously published in *The Journal of Child Psychotherapy*. Here we again see this innovative clinician sharing with us how he understands these difficult patients. He writes of therapeutic work offered both individually and in a group to patients who have turned to 'a mystical union with a bad object' which then gives rise to triumphant states of mind. He looks at the similarities between perversion and addiction and the fact that change can only come about 'once patients experience the anxieties at the basis of their addictions – the dreads that enactments protects them from'. Again, as throughout the book, we are seeing the belief that behaviour, that looked at from the outside seems to be 'perverse' and self-destructive, is in fact an attempted solution, a protection from anxieties that are experienced as overwhelming. This chapter also recognizes the usefulness of a group setting at times, work which is common for adult clinicians at the Portman, but less so for the child and adolescent psychotherapists. Through careful unravelling of the theory and brief descriptions of cases, Nathanson shows how, for the patients he is describing, 'a match is found between a specific unconscious dread and the way to triumph over it'. The chapter describes Nathanson's concept of the 'fuck it button', the moment when there is a transition from 'a state of passive suffering, not wanting to act, and a state of active excitement and omnipotence': this concept, only introduced in the last few years, has already become invaluable to clinicians. Nathanson describes painstakingly careful work which can enable the patient to slow down and see the moment of choice and take responsibility, develop a sense of separateness which diminishes their need to control the other, and loosens the grip of the 'cult' of the bad object.

The book closes with another brief chapter from Marianne Parsons detailing the history of the Portman Clinic in general and paying particular attention to the information that is in the archives about the sort of difficulties that brought people to the service over 75 years ago. Her roll call of the distinguished clinicians who have worked within the service make us, the more recent clinicians, very proud to be among their number The section on the historical reasons for referral is both fascinating and shocking: we are given a stark realization of how much society's attitudes have changed, how a moralistic approach, leaving little room for compassion or understanding pervaded. Her own clinical memories of the cases seen in the 1990s also gives an absorbing insight to more recent changes, and raises interesting questions about ways in which the patient population seems to have changed over time, especially the use of the Internet, pornography and social media.

This book integrates the experience of at least three generations of Portman clinicians. It is a group and tradition that we as editors are proud to belong to and currently represent. The Portman Clinic is an institution with a long history. As described in Parsons' chapter and by other researchers attending to this history elsewhere, it reflects cultural and social changes as much as it does psychoanalytic thinking and its special adaptation to the understanding of people who enact their difficulties by harming others, being delinquent and violent.

Working with children and young people within the context of a clinic treating adults, we can appreciate the way such disturbance starts early and develops through the full life-cycle. We also know from our work how our early interventions with young people can reroute a pathological trajectory, one psychologically engineered to survive early trauma, and open up a different trajectory, one harnessing the power of young people's psychic potential for emotional growth and development.

References

Balint, M. (1979) *The basic fault.* London/New York, Tavistock Publications.

Dockar-Drysdale, B. (1968) *Therapy in child care. Collected papers, etc.* United Kingdom, Longmans.

Golding, W (1954) *Lord of the flies.* London, Faber & Faber.

Glasser, M (1979) *Some aspects of the role of aggression in the perversions.* In: Rosen, I. (ed.) *Sexual deviations.* Oxford, OUP 1979.

King, D (2011) *Introduction in 'lord of the flies centenary edition'.* London, Penguin.

Rosenfeld, H. (1971) A clinical approach to the psychoanalytic theory of the life and death. *International Journal of Psycho-Analysis.* 52, 169–178.

Stoller, R. (1975) *Perversion: the erotic form of hatred.* New York, Pantheon.

Chapter 1

Key concepts developed at the Portman Clinic

Marianne Parsons

The Portman Clinic is a very special place. It is the only NHS institution where patients of all ages – children, adolescents and adults – who are delinquent, violent or suffering from sexual perversion are offered psychoanalytic psychotherapy to help them face and understand how and why they need to resort to using their bodies as an attempted 'solution' to unbearable feelings, fears and conflicts stemming from extremely traumatic past experiences. The clinicians aim to help the patients to begin to tolerate thinking about themselves rather than using action. In the case of children and adolescents, this way of thinking is also vital in working with the patient's carers and the professionals in the network, both in order to help them to understand better the internal forces propelling the youngster into unacceptable behaviours, and also to help them appreciate how they also may sometimes unwittingly jump into action with the patient and their colleagues out of their own anxiety and feelings of helplessness aroused by the case.

Child psychotherapists working at the Portman Clinic are in the privileged position of being highly valued by the adult psychotherapists and psychoanalysts, and presentations from members of the 'Child Team' at the Clinic's weekly discussion meetings have always been greatly appreciated. For clinicians working with adults, such presentations offer further insight into the developmental roots of disturbance in their patients.

Following Mervin Glasser's understanding of the global character structure of a perversion, (Glasser, 1986, 1992, 1996), which does not become fully established until adulthood, we don't consider children and adolescents with perverse behaviours as having a perversion because their development is still ongoing. Instead, they would be thought of as potentially on the way to developing a perversion. Providing skilled and sensitive therapy can help the young person's development to shift away from that trajectory and get back onto a more normative developmental track. This is also the aim with delinquent and violent patients.

At first, children and adolescents referred to the Clinic were seen by adult psychoanalysts, and it wasn't until the 1970s that the first qualified child and adolescent psychotherapist was employed. Over the ensuing years, this increased to two, three and then four clinicians dedicated to trying to understand the complex needs of young people who have no means other than via the use of their bodies to attempt to deal with the debilitating effects of extremely traumatic experiences in their early years. The Core Complex, Portman 'lore' and other thoughts on working with young people at the Portman Clinic are explained below.

The CORE COMPLEX is part of normative development in toddlerhood and is ultimately about difficulties with intimacy and separation, which we can all have to greater or lesser degrees – how to be with another without feeling taken over and controlled by the object and how to be separate without feeling utterly alone and empty. But for violent and perverse patients these anxieties are extremely intense and crippling. Glasser describes how such patients struggle to deal with the contrasting anxieties of being intruded upon, engulfed, overwhelmed and taken over by another on the one hand; and of being abandoned by the object, completely lost and alone on the other – i.e. too much or not enough closeness (intimacy). Underlying both anxieties is a primitive terror of annihilation – annihilation because of being taken over by another and therefore losing oneself, or annihilation because of being too separate and therefore feeling lost, abandoned and disintegrated. When feeling engulfed by another, the individual tries to protect himself by moving away from that person; but he[1] then experiences the opposite anxiety of being abandoned and alone, and so he moves towards the other again. This is an impossible situation and he swings back and forth between these two extremes, desperately trying to find a position of safety.

The Core Complex originates in the anal stage of pre-oedipal development outlined in the Freudian developmental model (Freud, A., 1972, 1976, 1992; Freud, S., 1905) where issues of separation–individuation, control and aggression are prominent and the dyadic relationship with the mother is most central. Typically, in the history of such patients, there is a mother whose narcissistic needs take precedence over her child's needs, so that the child cannot experience a safe emotional closeness with her and his capacity to develop a valued sense of himself as separate and different from her is severely compromised. Never feeling seen as himself, but only as a narcissistic extension of the mother, leads to extreme narcissistic vulnerability in the child and intense sensitivity to feelings of humiliation and helplessness. The lack of an emotionally available father further prevents the child from being able to experience a more healthy attachment relationship and find appropriate separateness from the damaging tie to a narcissistic mother.

Glasser emphasized the central role of aggression and its sexualization in this Core Complex dilemma: fear of the mother who is experienced as annihilatory (abandoning, engulfing, humiliating) arouses rage and an urge to destroy her, but there's also a desperate longing to reach her and a need to preserve her so as to be protected from abandonment and terrifying aloneness. Faced with the insoluble paradox of constantly trying to find a safe distance to preserve both the object and himself, he resorts unconsciously to sexualizing his aggression, i.e. sado-masochism. Sado-masochism (whether as a full sado-masochistic sexual perversion or a habitual way of relating without actual bodily expression) then becomes the attempted 'solution' used to defend against Core Complex anxieties. This enables the feared but much-needed object to be held onto at arm's length psychically – not too close or too distant – and safely in his control. Glasser contrasts sado-masochistic aggression with self-preservative aggression. Sado-masochistic aggression aims to maintain the tie (at a safe psychic distance) to the other, whereas self-preservative aggression aims to eliminate the other. If something breaks through the sado-masochistic defence, Core Complex anxieties and the ultimate terror of annihilation resurface in full force. The other is now perceived as threatening the survival of the Self, and so has to be destroyed. Self-preservative aggression then erupts in physical violence out of sheer panic for psychic survival. We would have a similar reaction if faced with a tiger in the jungle with no means of escape – we would want to kill it, not tease it.

In considering a sado-masochistic relationship, one can fall into the trap of seeing one person as the sadistic perpetrator who attacks and controls the other as the masochistic victim. However, one important element of what we call 'Portman lore' is that both parties can be sadistic as well as masochistic and both exert some control over the other. This way of thinking does not condone physical violence, of course, or lay blame on victims of abuse; it helps us to understand how violence becomes an integral part of a relationship which cannot exist without it. It also helps prevent the split of taking sides in relation to 'perpetrator' and 'victim', which often occurs in the professional network concerned with such cases, as both parties in such a scenario are understood as suffering from Core Complex anxieties, each with a mostly unconscious part to play in what happens.

Sado-masochism isn't only a habitual mode of relating between the individual and other people, but also features heavily in the interplay between parts of the patient's own mind. Due to early environmental impingements, these patients have a persecuting superego and an ego that isn't sufficiently developed to be able to process feelings and anxieties and protect the Self appropriately. With insufficient ego strength to intervene, the sadistic superego attacks and overwhelms the Self, humiliating and torturing it with its punitive 'voice'; but it also abandons the Self by allowing it no real self-esteem. This dynamic often reflects the child's experience of overpowering or neglectful parents, and the lack of any stable self-esteem is a characteristic of all Portman patients.

The intricacies of the Core Complex soon became central to the way Portman staff understood that any potentially intimate relationship, including that with the therapist, is a terrifying threat to their patients. This has huge implications for technique and requires very sensitive handling. If the stability of the patient's defensive sado-masochistic way of relating is threatened because he feels engulfed or abandoned by the therapist, or if his very fragile narcissism is undermined because he feels humiliated, the patient is likely to erupt in violent aggression as a kind of knee-jerk last-ditch attempt at psychic self-preservation. To avoid increasing the patient's anxieties and breaching their much-needed defences, we have to be extremely careful about what we say and especially how we say things, as the patient will so easily feel intruded upon, controlled, neglected, dismissed, humiliated and criticized.

Out of awareness of the patient's underlying Core Complex fears and the importance of respecting his need to keep at a safe-enough distance from the therapist, Portman staff always place the patient's chair rather than the therapist's nearest the door, to give the patient the security that he could escape if his anxiety became overwhelming, rather than needing to resort to physical attack on the therapist. Also, alarm buzzers were never introduced into consulting rooms at the Clinic, despite the fact that many risky patients were in therapy.

Unfortunately, this kind of psychoanalytic thinking has been replaced by action in many other settings today where risk is managed by the installation of alarm buzzers, glass screens and coded doors. This can lead patients to feel that their therapists perceive them as horribly dangerous and unbearable to be with, which is likely to arouse feelings of humiliation and fears of being taken over or abandoned, and so actually intensify the risk of their destructiveness.

Don Campbell candidly illustrates how he initially came to understand this with one of his first violent Portman adult patients, Mr D, who had been referred for habitually getting involved in pub fights after heavy drinking, often using broken bottles as weapons (Campbell, 2011). After discussing Mr D's early sessions with colleagues who asked if it was safe to have a glass ashtray within Mr D's reach, Don Campbell decided to remove the ashtray, but soon realized that this resort to action was a mistake. He had failed to recognize that the ashtray was an important potential weapon that enabled Mr D to feel safe in the presence of the analyst as a very dangerous transference figure. Removing the ashtray disarmed Mr D and 'increased his feelings of defencelessness'. This heightened his Core Complex terrors and actually put his analyst more at risk of Mr D's violence. Instead of feeling in the presence of someone strong and steady enough to help him, Mr D felt that his analyst was afraid of him and therefore wouldn't be able to see him as a whole person. Campbell reflected, 'By acting as I did ... I confirmed that I also dealt with my fears by resorting to action', and that 'I, like all the authorities he faced before, could not and would not think about his violence with him, but that I would have to do something about it. ... if I had thought more about the transference, and, especially, been more sensitive to my countertransference, I could have been more helpful' to Mr D (p. 4).

Child psychotherapists are trained to provide a box of toys appropriate for each patient, but before starting at the Portman I'd discovered the benefit of also having a cupboard in the room for general use containing play items for both boys and girls of all age groups. I'd been sharing a room with another child psychotherapist where there was such a toy cupboard, which I'd originally been very sniffy about, but it proved enormously helpful when I started seeing an 8-year-old boy whose mother worried about his aggressive outbursts at home and compulsive dressing-up in girls' clothes. He was very inhibited with me at first and resisted any fantasy play, but after a while he asked me to close my eyes and went to the big cupboard. Moments later, he told me to open my eyes and I saw a lace-gloved hand bedecked with plastic rings waving shyly at me as he hid behind the desk. From there on he used fantasy play with the 'girly' dressing-up things in the big cupboard to express his wish to be a girl and his conflicts about being a boy, which turned out to be about his fear of his aggression, terror of separating from his mum and anxiety about growing up. Towards the end of therapy, he pretended to be a young deer rubbing its head against a tree and told me with enormous pride that the antlers weren't fully grown yet, but each year they'd get bigger until he had ones like his dad! At the Portman, I introduced a similar cupboard for general use and it continued to be very useful there, for example with youngsters confused about their sexual identity and those who needed to have the opportunity to regress and express their more infantile needs through play, for example with dolls or a baby's bottle.

Play offers an arena for expressing feelings and experiences that cannot be put into words and where anxieties, fears and urges that would otherwise be enacted with the body can be displaced safely. With all children, but especially those with Core Complex anxieties, it is important to be engaged with and share the child's play, but not to intrude by interpreting potential underlying meanings too early. Otherwise, the child's Core Complex anxieties will be intensified because of feeling threatened by an abandoning or engulfing object. Allowing the play to unfold at its own pace gives the child the experience of being with a different kind of object with whom a different way of relating may become possible. The child may now be able to experience their previously unmet needs for concern for their well-being and appropriate care and attentiveness being met by the therapist as a new developmental object (Hurry, 1998).

What applies to playing with younger children also applies to the way of listening to and talking with older children and adolescents. Tom, aged 17, instigated violent fights with boys and had attempted to rape a girl at knifepoint. He found it very hard to be in the room with me and would stare silently at me with a penetrating gaze, which felt both intrusive and dismissive;

but underneath his intimidating stare I sensed his fear of me. He wanted me to ask questions but would then feel intruded upon, and if I stayed silent, he seemed to experience me as not being interested or bothered about him. This made his Core Complex dilemma very clear – he felt both engulfed and abandoned by me, and I felt similarly in relation to him. Eventually I said that I had a dilemma to think about with him – that I thought my words as well as my silence made him feel awful, and he seemed to feel very unsafe and un-comfortable in the room with me. As I tried to explore his discomfort with me, it emerged that he found all verbal communication difficult. He felt he had nothing interesting to say and that nobody noticed him. I said that must make him feel terribly lonely and it might be very hard for him to feel he was a 'somebody' worthy of notice. Perhaps it was as if he felt invisible? He agreed and said that the only thing that would always make people pay attention to him was when he talked about his racist political opinions. It didn't matter whether the person agreed or disagreed, all that mattered was to get an intense reaction. I linked this urgent need to get through to people with his helpless isolation of never having felt noticed in a good way by his parents, especially his mother. I wondered if the only way he felt he could make an impact on someone was by force – by his forceful political views or physical violence. This seemed to reach him, and he responded thoughtfully by saying for the first time that he felt helpless and vulnerable sometimes. Tom had built a pseudo-identity as a 'tough guy' to protect himself from feeling vulnerable to humiliation, abandonment and intrusiveness. With violent and negating parents and no age-appropriate allowance for omnipotence in early child-hood, the smallest humiliation was experienced by Tom as the most terrible trauma. Underneath the presentation of himself as an all-powerful young man, there was a frightened and humiliated child whose only way of pro-tecting himself from an overwhelming sensitivity to feeling a rejected nobody was to act violently. Coldly calculated violence shaped Tom's identity so that he could try to avoid dealing with terrifying Core Complex anxieties and therefore would not experience the ultimate threats to his psychic survival (Parsons, 2009).

When a patient was referred, be it for a risk assessment, consultation for the professional network, a court report or as a potential psychotherapy patient, we sought all possible material on the patient and often ended up with a massive amount of reports, some of which had missed out vital details of the patient's history. One of the most important first tasks was to compile a detailed and comprehensive background history of the patient to ensure that we got as full a picture as possible of the patient's development and to ensure that important facts or events did not get lost. This is in itself could often help professionals when we also offered psychoanalytic understanding in ordinary language about how the patient's offending behaviour was their attempted unconscious 'solution' to the terrors, anxieties and conflicts in their internal world.

When patients came for an assessment, they were usually extremely resistant and anxious, even if they tried to cover up their fear by apparent bravado, as they seemed convinced that they would be perceived only as 'bad' because of their problematic behaviours. One adolescent boy said later in therapy that it was as if he had 'child abuser' tattooed on his forehead. It is vital to help the youngster to see that we can appreciate their positive characteristics and that we don't only focus on their problems. Because of their traumatic experiences and the lack of good-enough care in their early years, their emotional development had been stunted and skewed, and so, as Anna Freud noted in writing about very aggressive children, the 'appropriate therapy (has) to be directed to the neglected, defective side, ie the emotional libidinal development' (Freud, 1949). To foster this development and enhance the youngster's self-esteem and capacity to be curious about himself, it is of vital importance to help him to feel seen by the therapist as a whole person with strengths that can be valued (as well as weaknesses that need help). This offers hope to the patient and is essential for a move towards a healthier future.

Note

1 For the sake of brevity, 'he' will be used to cover patients of both genders.

References

Campbell, D. (2011) The nature and function of aggression. In: Williams, P.(ed.) *Aggression: from fantasy to action*. London, Karnac Books. pp. 1–15.

Freud, A. (1949) Aggression in relation to emotional development: normal and pathological. In: *The writings of Anna Freud*. Vol. 4. New York, International Universities Press. pp. 489–497.

Freud, A. (1972) The widening scope of psychoanalytic child psychology: normal and abnormal. In: *The writings of Anna Freud*. Vol. 8. New York, International Universities Press. pp. 8–33.

Freud, A. (1976) Psychopathology seen against the background of normal development. In: *The writings of Anna Freud*. Vol. 8. New York, International Universities Press. pp. 82–95.

Freud, A. (1992) Lecture five: stages of development. In: Sandler, J. (ed.) *The Harvard lectures*. London, Karnac Books.

Freud, S. (1905) Three essays on the theory of sexuality. In: Strachey, J. (transl. and editor) *The standard edition of the complete psychological works of Sigmund Freud*. SE VII. 24 vols. London: Hogarth Press and the Institute of Psychoanalysis, 1953.

Glasser, M. (1986) Identification and its vicissitudes as observed in the perversions. *The International Journal of Psychoanalysis*. 67, 9–16.

Glasser, M. (1992) Problems in the psychoanalysis of certain narcissistic disorders. *The International Journal of Psychoanalysis*. 73, 493–503.

Glasser, M. (1996) Aggression and sadism in the perversion. In: Rosen, I. (ed.) Sexual deviation. 3rd ed. Oxford, OUP.

Hurry, A. (1998) Psychoanalysis and developmental therapy. In: Hurry, A. (ed.) *Psychoanalysis and developmental therapy*. London, Karnac. pp. 32–73.

Parsons, M. (2009) The roots of violence: theory and implications for technique with children and adolescents. In: Lanyado, M. & Horne, A. (eds.) *The handbook of child and adolescent psychotherapy*. Revised edition. London, Routledge.

Chapter 2

Motiveless malignity: problems in the psychotherapy of patients with psychopathic features

Anne Alvarez

Introduction

This chapter explores the difficult issue of how to understand – and meet – the very particular nature of the destructiveness of the psychopathic child. I draw attention to the difference between the state of mind and inner world of the neurotic, borderline and psychopathic patient, with reference to different types of destructiveness: anger in the neurotic patient; desperate vengeful hatred in the borderline paranoid and a cold addiction to violence in the psychopath. I will discuss technical issues and the need to meet the psychopathic patient where he really is, in the inner bleak emotional cemetery he may inhabit. Honest and brave description of what we are seeing, however costly to therapeutic zeal, seems far more effective than attempts to explain (and thus seem to explain away) the destructive behaviour. Needless to say, the patients themselves refuse to stay put in the neat schematic categories I have outlined; but they do seem to appreciate our recognizing the specific quality of these vastly different states of mind. The Portman Child and Adolescent Psychotherapists have developed real expertise with these sorts of patients – they are capable of great tact, humour, respect and fearlessness, and I'm honoured to have my thoughts included in their book.

A film called *Assault on Precinct 13* begins with a sequence of shots of a gang of young men riding around the Watts District of Los Angeles in a car, aiming rifles first at an old black woman, then at a white man, then at a black man. Their fun is at least racially undiscriminating. The aiming seems random, idle, almost whimsical. We get to see the quarry lined up in the sights of the rifle each time, but no one pulls the trigger. The members of the gang seem to be having a good time (Bruce Chatwin observed that in the language of many nomadic peoples, the word for townspeople is 'meat' (1987)). The scene then switches to a little girl buying an ice cream from an ice cream vendor while her father makes a phone call from a call box. She returns to her father, but suddenly looks at her ice cream with dismay and turns back to the ice cream van. She does not realize that by then the gang has killed the ice cream vendor, and the man standing in the van is his killer.

She says, 'Excuse me, I asked for chocolate and you've given me strawberry!' The killer turns and, as casually as he might swat a fly, shoots her in her still open mouth. It is horrifying, and what is particularly horrifying about it is the casualness. The killer does not appear to be angry, nor does he give any sign of sadistic relish. He looks at most mildly irritated.

In another film, *House of Games* by David Mamet, a con-man tricks his woman psychiatrist out of all her savings. At first, she – and we – are led to think he is in love with her. In fact, he is a member of a group of con-men. When she learns of her seduction and betrayal, she speaks of their love affair and asks, outraged, disbelieving, and hurt, 'How could you do that to me?' He says, calmly, and with a dismissive shrug, 'But this is what I do'.

Psychoanalysts and psychiatrists have described the lack of conscience in psychopaths, the lack of guilt and remorse for their deeds, their indifference to their victims' cries for mercy. The more modern psychiatric classifications have tried to avoid what had in part become the pejorative and wastebasket use of the term 'psychopath', but the newer terms – 'conduct disorder', 'antisocial personality disorder', even 'sociopath' have become inadequate, because their purely descriptive level of meaning does not distinguish between the kind of destructiveness which is motivated by anger, that by bitter hatred, that by outrage, that by sadism, and that by casual brutality.

This has been even more true in the field of Child Psychiatry: this is beginning to change, however, at least in the child psychiatric research. Viding has suggested that psychopathy should be seen as a developmental disorder (2004), and Frick and White have reviewed the research on the importance of callous-emotional personality traits for a particular sub-group of anti-social and aggressive youth (2008). Unlike the previous textbooks, the research shows that the youths themselves know it is not a simple question of anger. Indeed, they seem comfortable with their lack of empathy (Frick & White, 2008). The review suggests that making these distinctions is important for treatment, but it is not clear what treatment they consider might reach such children. Certainly, motivated vengeful paranoid violence is different from addictive habitual violence. Addictive violence may have begun as a defence against some horror, then gradually acquired sadistic and exciting overtones, but eventually, under certain conditions of lifelong chronicity, become almost motiveless and certainly casual. The enormity of the act may no longer bear any relation to the amount of feeling left in the perpetrator. An addiction is different from a defence. A temporary defensive hardening of the heart is different from a lifelong arteriosclerosis of the emotions. A big freeze is different from a brief chill.

A child with psychopathic features

My own school of hard knocks began with a little girl called Sarah. She was a destructive and violent child who regularly used to attack me physically.

When she threw chairs at me in Friday sessions, I would say, 'You are beating me up today because it's the weekend and we have to say goodbye and you don't like being left'. She would agree, 'Yes' and then she would kick me again. I would make a similar interpretation on Monday, 'You are kicking me because I left you on the weekend'. Gradually I began to think, 'but she kicks me on Tuesday and Wednesday and Thursday too!' She simply *liked* kicking people. She had, I learned belatedly, a strong sado-masochistic element in her personality. After some years of the physical violence, she moved to mental cruelty. She knew how to interrupt, with impeccable, almost musical timing, at exactly the moment when I was about to get something important finally formulated and clear. She knew how to raise hopes and then dash them. It was high art, and her concentration was dedicated, precise, and unremitting. If she tried to fly a paper butterfly, and it sank, she would turn at the first second of its failure, and sneer, 'You thought it was going to fly, didn't you?' In fact, she too had thought for a moment that it would fly, but the hope got projected so instantaneously, and then destroyed so equally instantaneously, that it required, not simply careful monitoring on my part on a moment-by-moment basis, but *second-by-second* monitoring. I often complained to any colleague who would listen, that no-one who had not spent a lifetime's *practice*, as my patient had, in defeating herself and others, could possibly keep up with such a person. I felt I did care about monitoring our interactions on a moment-by-moment basis, but I wasn't even sure that I *wanted* to be vigilant in such micro-analytic terms, from second to second. Betty Joseph's (1989) writings were helpful in discouraging the superficial use of explanatory interpretations with borderline patients. Her teachings and writings on ad-dictive processes were indispensable (1982). Also, Herbert Rosenfeld sug-gested to me that Bion's dictum of shedding memory and desire was not appropriate with such patients. On the contrary, he thought one needed to be very vigilant, and always a step ahead, because otherwise they despised you. (Certainly, they seem to be wonderfully alert to hypocrisy). I would agree with Rosenfeld, as far as the psychopathic part of the patient is concerned, and shall suggest that, long before goodness is at issue, such patients are mea-suring us for our courage, strength and inability to be fooled. (Their des-pairing and persecuted parts may, however, require other tender – rather than tough-minded sensibilities of us.) These patients are probably at the schizoid end of what Melanie Klein (1935) called the paranoid/schizoid – depressive continuum, and for the most hardened or grandiose ones, becoming paranoid and persecuted is actually sometimes something of a development. When, instead of feeling no concern for themselves, they begin to fear retribution, this, strangely enough, can signal a reduction in grandiosity or at least a melting of the emotional ice. The internal object may have begun to take on a little substantiality and life, even if only of a dangerous kind. An object somewhere has become capable of witnessing, and taking seriously, the danger to the self. At least something matters. (Clearly, this is nowhere near the depressive position in terms of concern for others; nevertheless, developments within the paranoid position remain developments and should not be discounted simply because they do not involve depressive position concern or guilt.) It is interesting that when the psychopathic killer in the film *No Country for Old Men* comes, at the end of the film, to kill the woman who is the wife and daughter of his two previous victims, he seems surprised at her refusal to let him flip a coin, which if it falls right, could save her life. She is different from all his previous victims, who either fought back pathetically, begged, or tried to bargain for their life. She, in contrast, simply looks at him steadily, waiting for him to kill her. We are spared her murder, but in the next scene, he is seen driving down her road, looking in the rear view mirror as two boys clown about on their bikes behind him. He seems rattled by them, and in the only moment in the film where he loses control, he crashes the car and injures himself badly. I think he was rattled by her bleak courage.

Some clinical differentiation between neurotic, borderline and psychopathic states of mind

I would like now to differentiate first, anger in a neurotic patient; second, desperation, outrage and vengeance in two borderline patients; and third, icy calculating cruelty in a very young psychopathic patient. I shall then consider four technical issues in the treatment of psychopathic patients. Of course, as I have said previously, live human beings refuse to stay put in these neat schematic categories, and I am using these diagnostic categories for purposes of discussion only. I have also become interested in recent years in the element of psychopathy or personality disorder in some children with autism, an issue that requires more space to discuss (Alvarez, 1999; Alvarez & Lee, 2004).

I have given an example in *The Thinking Heart* (Alvarez, 2012: p.14) with a neurotic patient, where more ordinary interpretations about anger due to loss or jealousy were possible. She was functioning at a relatively well neurotic level, where it can be positively helpful to say something like, 'You are cross, you are angry because...'. This is in patients where there is some capacity for guilt, some capacity for love, some ego which can process insight into their own aggression, but also, some already established self-respect so they can bear to face hurt and frustration

Borderline patients

A different situation arose with a little boy called Peter whose therapist who was leaving the Clinic in a month's time. He came to his session in a very desperate, wild, fragmented state. His mother, who, like him, was upset about the ending and unable to acknowledge it, had taken to bringing him late. He had a very deprived first year of his life, when his (anyway) rather withdrawn mother was very profoundly depressed. After a few minutes, he took out a paper with a calendar of their sessions, asking when they would be stopping and which was today. His therapist offered to tick off the days, something they had recently stopped doing. He said 'No' and started to tear up the calendar. The therapist said that Peter was cross with her about their meetings stopping (i.e. 'angry because' – an explanatory defence interpretation). Peter got wilder and overturned a chair; she tried to prevent him and again said that he was angry because they were stopping the meetings. He began to get even more excited, banging his head against the wall, something he did regularly as a baby. Here I think it is not enough to interpret anger. There is despair, and the child's desperate impotence and helplessness may be increased and escalated unhelpfully at such moments. He is incapable of hearing it, because he is in no fit state to think about and process anger. The necessary ego functioning and the necessary hope are both lacking. Yet, if the therapist is willing to take some of the badness in to herself or himself, the child may begin to find things slightly more bearable, and to process the experience. So one might say something like (with some feeling, by the way): 'It's really *terrible* for you that I'm stopping. You feel you should be able to tear this whole experience up. It *shouldn't* be happening, I *shouldn't* be leaving you'. This would involve acknowledging the child's desperation and amplifying and carrying for him his as yet unnamed, unverbalized, but possibly at least 'pre-conceived' (Bion, 1962) sense of injustice. (See Alvarez, 1999; Alvarez & Lee, 2004 for a fuller discussion of the issue of responding to moral imperatives.) I should also mention the importance of recognizing that some traumatized children act impulsively in states of PTSD and need to be shown that we recognize that it is 'in them to do' which is different from the assumption that they own what they are doing. Violence can erupt as a result of abuse or of witnessing violence, and the child may rightly feel that he didn't mean to do it, someone else did it.

In patients who are more paranoid, phantasies, not acts, of others getting deserved punishment – that is, phantasies of justice and revenge – may enable desperate and needed projections to occur and be contained. Joseph (1978) discusses the dangers of premature return of projections with borderline patients. The relieving calming effect seems to have to do with an understanding that badness needs to *stay out there*. Otherwise, humiliation, despair, shame and revenge can lead to explosive and dangerous eruptions in patients who may have been very heavily projected into. This kind of desperate, embittered hatred has to be carefully distinguished from the aggression of the more casually brutal, or more coldly murderous psychopath who, of course, could experience the above interpretations as collusion.

Patients with psychopathic features

Hyatt Williams (1998) has pointed out that if one worked very carefully with murderers with an adequate theory of splitting, displacement and projection, it was possible to discover that they were not without conscience: they did have a conscience but only in regard to particular split-off objects. For example, a man who had murdered a woman might not feel guilty about the woman, but might suddenly feel pity and remorse for an injured pigeon. Symington (1980) makes the similar point, that if you look carefully at the internal world of these people, they do have a good object and love for it somewhere, but it is often invisible and hidden. They are not completely conscienceless, not completely loveless. They have an excess of guilt. He cites Heathcliff's symbiotic love for Catherine in Emily Bronte's novel, *Wuthering Heights* (1847). I would stress that what also kept Heathcliff going was his belief in her love of him. In some of the colder psychopathic people, however, it would be hard to find even that bit of light in the darkness. Meloy (1996) a psychologist who has had a long and intensive experience with violent inmates in prisons in the San Diego area in California, has made a very helpful distinction between what he calls 'affectively evoked aggression' – aggression evoked by the perception of threat and 'predatory aggression' – which is directed towards the destruction of prey, usually for food-gathering in sub-human species. It involves minimal autonomic arousal and vocalization.

> When a household cat is cornered and threatened, the neurochemical set produces a display of affective aggression: hissing, hair standing on end, dilating pupils, active clawing arching back. When the same cat is stalking a bird in the back-yard, predatory aggression dominates: quiet stalking of the prey, the absence of ritualistic display, and focussed attention on the target.

He states that predatory aggression is the hallmark of the psychopath. (He is careful to distinguish between the severe and mild ends of a continuum of psychopathy, and thinks people from the milder end tend to be treatable.) Meloy suggests that the anecdotal descriptions (1996:p.74) by workers in forensic treatment and custody settings of certain patients or inmates eyes as 'cold, staring, harsh, empty, vacant and absent of feeling' and the consequent feeling of eerie fear should be taken very seriously. He points out that this experience of chilling fear does not seem to arise with even very dangerous explosive combative patients.

Technical problems with patients with psychopathic features

I want now to draw attention to a major theme in Symington's (1980) paper: his brilliant delineation of the three responses evoked by the psychopath. He points out that one of the most common responses is collusion. People simply let bullies have what they want. He suggests that this has something to do with gratification of some of our own psychopathic parts. He says that the second common response is disbelief and denial. I think it is possible, but useless or dangerous, to use psychoanalytic explanation both to the patient and to ourselves in exactly this denying way, in order to evade the disturbing facts of what we are feeling in the counter-transference. And these patients know when we are being evasive and cannot stand what they are dishing out. Symington is quite forgiving about the fear such people evoke in their analysts, therapists, or jailers, and the naturalness of our cowardly denials. He points out that it is only sane to want safety and peace. The third response is condemnation. These patients do provoke the most powerful feelings of horror, outrage, condemnation and retaliation. Unfortunately, such responses only serve to excite the patient, or make him strengthen his armoury and become even more determined to defeat you. The hardest thing to do is really to look evil in the eye, bravely but not in a retaliatory or condemnatory way. When I finally became aware of how much Sarah relished putting the knife in and then twisting it, I was at first shocked and horrified. I would say, 'You really want to break my heart, don't you?' I suspect my use of the word 'really' still carried a note of disbelief, and the vain hope that she would deny it. Instead, she would lean forward intently and whisper – fervently – 'Yes!' I think if you work with these patients for any length of time you have to grow and change because they change you. One has to get beyond the stage of denial, then beyond the state of outrage to a state of mind requiring courage and steadfastness, and also, in one sense, respect for the patient's courage in surviving in his empty world.

I wanted to say something about a book by Docker-Drysdale (1990), a follower of Winnicott who ran a residential unit for extremely disturbed children. She wrote about 'frozen' children who, I think, may be even more ill than Heathcliff and the people that Symington was talking about. I think we have to leave room in our minds for the fact that some children get frozen so early in life that there isn't a lot of love even hidden. Docker-Drysdale makes it clear that she would always be looking for some flicker of feeling in assessing a child for acceptance into the school. She wrote most interestingly about the difficulty these children have with symbolization. She gives an example of a child new to the school who may steal from the refrigerator, not because the food has any symbolic meaning, but simply because he's hungry. A couple of years later, when the child is by now very attached to his primary care worker, he may steal from the refrigerator because he is upset because she is going on holiday: the theft may be full of symbolic meaning. Docker-Drysdale thinks it is important not to confuse the two. Hanna Segal's (1957) distinction between the symbolic equation and the true symbol are relevant here, as is Winnicott's (1953) concept of the transitional phase. It is fascinating to watch these children move from vicious acting out, to played viciousness, to, say, a cruel verbal joke, and then to a kinder joke, a progressive process which may take months or years but which is nevertheless an important development involving some considerable sparing of the object.

Docker-Drysdale thinks that such children are 'unable to make any real object relationships or to feel the need for them'. And, importantly, 'This kind of child cannot symbolize what he has never experienced or realized' (p.179). In the same way, I am suggesting that it is important to find a language sufficiently bleak for the psychopath to feel we are at least attempting to meet him where he really is, rather than where we think he ought to be. In a large part of his being, he may inhabit an emotional cemetery. We can neither exhort nor coax him into the depressive position, and to join the rest of the human race. He will only think we are misguided fools if we talk to him about the anger or loss or pain which he may be years away from feeling. Nor should we imagine he is necessarily defending himself against dependency on us, or refusing to see our goodness. He may really see us as useless, because he has a useless internal object. His violence may have begun as a defence against pain, but it may have changed into a way of life.

Docker-Drysdale made an interesting distinction between experience, realization and symbolization: she pointed out that it is not enough to give these children good experiences; they have to realize they're having them. This is similar to my own views derived from working with very deprived or very abused children. You may need to interpret when you see that, for example, 'You feel that I like you today' or 'You like me today' but you also need to begin to show them that they *like* being liked, they *like* having loving feelings. 'You like to please me, and you like it when I like you'. These children are often caught up in a vicious circle in which they do something provocative, the object punishes, they then do something even more provocative, and they may rarely notice the other, probably very fleeting moments of good contact. (Such interpretations might need to be even cooler and more matter-of-fact with patients in a psychopathic state.)

Docker-Drysdale's concept of realization is similar both to Bion's (1962) concept of the need to get 'alpha function' around a thought to make it thinkable and developmental theories of how experience acquires meaning. Stern (1985) was describing a rather more pleasant set of meanings than was Bion, whereas here the experience we are invited – or rather forced – to share or contain is disturbing and often horrifying, and it is easy to miss tiny reductions in the level of cruelty, for example, or fleeting moments of friendliness. But when these moments come, we can learn not to greet them too eagerly, and not to make too fancy symbolic explanatory interpretations. It seems better simply to stay with the patient and think about one moment of his experience at a time. With psychopaths, Strachey's (1934) concept of 'minimal doses' in the transference probably needs reducing to 'minimalistic doses'. These people often hate any comment too heavy with meaning, because it is felt to be therefore too laden with emotion, and a lifetime of dissociation has led to emotion being seen as loathsome, contemptible or irrelevant.

A second example of a child with psychopathic features: Billy

Sarah, whom I mentioned earlier, was only 10 years old, and it was originally hard to believe that such a young child could be capable of such dedication to cruelty. Subsequently, I treated a little four-year-old boy whom I shall call Billy; referred because of his coldness to his mother. (His mother believed the child had never looked at her since he was born. In fact, the mother was rarely at home, and the child became profoundly attached to his Nanny, who then left and was replaced by a series of different nannies.) At one point, Billy became very withdrawn, but both before and after this period, he had hardened up chillingly. He was an attractive child, who could charm strangers with his intelligence and lively, rather driven sense of drama, but he developed an icy glitter, and a manipulativeness which worried even his father, who did not feel rejected by him. Billy was extremely jealous of and cruel to, his younger more favoured two-year-old sister, and in his sessions, he indulged in slow, calculated tortures performed by a 'doctor' (himself) on a toy baby teddy. I was instructed to speak for the teddy, and, obviously losing my capacity to bear it at one point one day, I made the mistake of asking, in the teddy's voice, why I was receiving such punishment, why the doctor was doing this to me. He looked at me as though I was utterly stupid, and replied, 'Why? Because I like it!' I had seen him a day or so before sticking the pin of his badge into the teddy's eyes, infinitely slowly and with almost loving relish, and I should have known better. Terms such as 'conduct disorder' do not capture the flavour of such moments. Such destructiveness is different in kind from impulsive anger or fury: it feels lifelong, abiding, enduring and, even in a four-year old, lifelong means just that – his life of bitter disappointment had been inordinately long.

I usually did not refer to the teddy as representing his own baby part, or to infantile dependency feelings being spared. At times it was filled with otherness, and represented, I think, his hated little sister. I believe the desire, and in a way, as Kundera suggests, the *need* for rectifying revenge phantasies (not actions) may need addressing for a very long period. The clinician has to decide when the patient is able to accept the return of the split-off or projected part. This may be a few seconds, or a few years later. The clinician also has to try and sense when violence has become somewhat desultory and is also no longer needed. Billy had genuine borderline paranoid features, but these were beginning to solidify into something more psychopathic.

Billy's parents were never sure at that stage that psychotherapy was what they wanted for him, and it became clear that as he had become more manageable, his treatment would have to end. He was also less withdrawn and that seemed to be enough for them. The Monday after the weekend when they had rung to confirm their decision that he should stop at Easter, he came into his session in a bullying but blustering and wild state. First he blocked my path on the stairs down to the playroom. I said it seemed to be my turn to be shut out. Then in, for him, a very muddled way, (he was usually icily clear and coherent) he began to say, 'They say I am not coming – they asked me what I... I don't want to come here anymore. No... they don't want... No... I don't want...' I said I thought he was muddled, because he wasn't sure who it was who didn't want him to come. He kept on repeating, as he opened his case, 'I don't want to come any more – you're a.... bad witch'. Yet although at one point he was facing me, and normally he has the boldest of un-childlike gazes, this time he would not look at my face. Instead, he was staring down somewhere around my middle. I said I thought he was having difficulty looking at me and maybe this was because he wasn't sure what he wanted and whether I really was all bad. He began throwing all his toys out of his box onto the floor, but when he got to the bottom layer, which contained the farm and wild animals, he first took out the little lamb, placed it carefully inside a glove puppet and placed a white and brown foal in front, as though to stand guard over it. They had been good figures guarding the little lamb the week before, and I was surprised at their survival. He went on with terrible and final deliberation, throwing all the other animals out on the floor with total contempt, and grinding his feet slowly and thoroughly onto the soft baby rabbit. He seemed too wound up and icy even to get into one of his sadistic 'games' with me where the animals were to be killed and eaten. His contempt (and, I think, his despair) was too total even to play. I acknowledged this, but I did comment on the lamb's preservation. I said I thought that he was leaving a little room in his mind for friendly feelings and some good memories of the time he'd spent here. I kept it cool and minimalistic, as I believe was right with him. It saved his dignity and in a way acknowledges his courage in the enormity of his task, which involved managing his own enormous hatred and the hatred, which he felt others had for him. I did not, therefore, refer to a baby part, or to infantile dependency feelings being spared. A little later, he shouted, 'You'll be sorry!', and I, feeling absolutely terrible anyway, said I thought he felt I should be the one to feel the sadness about his going. And that maybe he knew I *was* very sad, and didn't want to lose him. After a bit, I added that he must feel I ought to be sorry about not being strong enough to have persuaded his parents to let him stay. He began to glance at me a little. He began to order me, in a very tyrannical manner, to pick up the fallen toys. I felt the situation was mixed because he was a tyrannical child, and the services he got people to perform in this way were invariably done grudgingly, if not with hatred. But I also felt he was getting more and more desperate, and that he actually needed me to pick the things up, and to show that I was willing to do it because I liked him, not forced to do it because I feared his tantrums. Also, he was finally engaging me in a joint activity, in however bullying a manner. So I began to pick the things up, keeping my eyes on him, which was hard to do when he was glaring so unpleasantly and coldly. I think he was certain, as all tyrants are, that his slaves hated him.

There was a noise from upstairs in the house, and he startled very suddenly. I said that I thought that he was afraid somebody up there didn't like him bullying me like this, and that he felt I really didn't like him when he ordered me around like this. (My years of incomprehension and denial with Sarah may have taught me something, because I did say this with great seriousness, but note the 'really'.) He started to say, 'I don't want to come here', but it came out, 'You don't want to come here' and eventually I said, making myself look at him, realizing that there was truth in it, 'I think you feel I'm glad you're going'. He gave me a very direct look.

Note that I did not say, 'You are afraid that I'm glad you're going', as the verb containing doubt – 'afraid that' – can serve to deny what is really happening between the patient's self and his object. It is important to contain the reality of his emotional experience, and the word 'feel' is less denying. (See Winnicott, 1947, on hate in the countertransference.) Looking the patient in the eye bravely means also having the courage to look at oneself honestly.

When it was time to go, he shouted on the stairs up, 'How would YOU like it if you had to be put in a box!', and I had just time to say that I thought he felt really it ought to be me and not him that this was happening to. I let him know I thought he was right, because it seemed that this time it was a desperate, not a cruel projective identification. In fact, I think on reflection that it was not even a projective identification, more an acknowledgement of his failure to project, his inability to find and keep an object that could receive his projections. He now rarely saw the beloved nanny of the past, and I think he was describing his own fate as the receiver of his mother's powerful projections. But the further element in his question, which I could not address in the month remaining to us before the termination of treatment was, 'Do you really care to know in full what it's like to be me?' I suspect Billy knew that a part of me did not.

Discussion and conclusion: four technical issues

I would like to conclude by discussing four issues, which arise in working with such patients. In order to avoid Symington's trio of collusion, denial and condemnation, it is important first, to avoid the last: that is, instead of condemnation, it is necessary to look evil straight in the eye. This implies not evading the full bleakness and horror of the patient's impulses, nor the inadequacy and foolishness of their internal objects and of ourselves in the transference. As the doctor–torturer–child replied to me, 'I like it!' It also implies not evading what they know to be our own dislike, distaste and even hatred for their ruthless, cruel and often brutal treatment of us, their objects and themselves. I don't know if I have conveyed the degree to which Billy's play with the baby teddy was not simply ordinary aggressive phantasied play, or why I feel that he was the kind of child who might really have caused an accident to his baby sister, so carefully managed that no one would ever know that it was anything but an accident.

There was, however, also a desperate paranoid element, and it was important that someone receive the projections which no-one had been able to hold, and to be honest about what he knew to be his object's hatred and weariness. Hopefully, one could do this without retaliation. Unfortunately, there was the further problem that his cruelty was becoming the possible grounding for a sado–masochistic perversion. He 'trembled' with excitement in some of his scenes. This certainly needed addressing in later intensive work with him, which was eventually carried out with considerable success.

Second, we must struggle not to collude or deny, but to find, unsentimentally, the patient's friendly feelings and whatever faint beginnings there may be of trust and faith. We should not appeal for a good self or good object which is not present, but we need to be alert to the tiniest flickerings of faith and hope that are there. It is dangerous to elevate or amplify them; it is better by far to play them down. The patient may be able to agree that he is somewhat irritated at the recent break's interruption to his routine, but be nowhere near getting in touch with painful feelings of loss about the gap. Also, at times we may have to acknowledge, unsentimentally, what he may observe to be our hurt, our defeat, and our fondness when the patient cannot do so.

Third, it is usually important to avoid symbolic interpretations of either positive or negative feelings. For example, interpretations along the lines of, 'You feel abandoned by me as you did by your mother' may carry too much meaning, and meaning may simply not be available to patients in these hardened frozen states. We may need to respect the patient's insistence that he 'just' likes what he does, or 'just' is irritated, not angry today, and that it has no meaning. Then, slowly – perhaps – meaning can grow.

Finally, two-part interpretations directed towards searching out and revealing the patient's vulnerability are usually dangerous or useless. Such patients are not functioning at the level of the depressive position. They are living in a paranoid world where survival, not love, is at issue. Values of intelligence, daring, courage, skill, triumph – the values of the battlefield – are paramount. Premature interpretations regarding hidden vulnerability or dependence, which the patient has not yet owned, may produce dangerous eruptions, or, at the very least, earn the patient's appropriate contempt. It is important, instead, to save his dignity and respect his courage in going on in the face of the dead world he inhabits.

References

Alvarez, A. (1999) Addressing the deficit: developmentally informed psychotherapy with passive, 'undrawn' children. In: Alvarez, A. & Reid, S. (eds.) *Autism and personality: findings from the Tavistock autism workshop*. London, Routledge.

Alvarez, A. (2012) *The thinking heart*. London & New York, Routledge.

Alvarez, A. & Lee, A. (2004) Early forms of relatedness in autism. *Clinical Child Psychology and Psychiatry*. 9 (4), 499–518.

Bion, W. R. (1962) *Learning from experience*. London, Heinemann.

Bronte, E. (1965) *Wuthering heights* (1847). Harmondsworth, Penguin.

Chatwin, B. (1987) *The songlines*. London, Jonathon Cape.

Docker-Drysdale, B. (1990) *The provision of primary experience: Winnicottian work with children and adolescents*. London, Free Association Books.

Frick, P. J. & White, S. F. (2008) Research review: the importance of callous-unemotional traits for developmental models of aggressive and antisocial behaviour. *Journal of Consulting and Clinical Psychology*. 49 (4), 359–375.

Hyatt Williams, A. (1998) *Cruelty, violence and murder*. London, Karnac Books.

Joseph, B. (1978) Different types of anxiety and their handling in the clinical situation. In: Spillius, E. B. & Feldman, M. (eds.) (1989) *Psychic equilibrium and psychic change: selected papers of Betty Joseph*. London, Routledge.

Joseph, B. (1982) Addiction to near death. In: Spillius, E. B. & Feldman, M. (eds.) (1989) *Psychic equilibrium and psychic change: selected papers of Betty Joseph*. London, Routledge.

Klein, M. (1935) A contribution to the psychogenesis of manic depressive states. In: Khan, M. Masud R. (ed.). *The writings of Melanie Klein, volume III Melanie Klein: envy and gratitude and other works* (1975). London, Hogarth.

Kundera, M. (1982) *The joke*. Harmondsworth, Middlesex, Penguin Books.

Meloy, J. R. (1996) *The psychopathic mind: origin, dynamics, treatment*. London, Jason Aronson.

Segal, H. (ed.) (1957) Notes on symbol formation. In: *The work of Hanna Segal*, 1981. New York, Aronson.

Stern, D. (1985) *The interpersonal world of the infant*. New York, Basic Books.

Strachey, J. (1934) The nature of the therapeutic action of psychoanalysis. *International Journal of Psychoanalysis*. 15, 127–159.

Symington, N. (1980) The response aroused by the psychopath. *International Review of Psychoanalysis*. 7, 291–298.

Viding, E. (2004) Annotation: understanding the development of psychopathy. *Journal of Child Psychology and Psychiatry*. 45 (8) 1329–1337.

Winnicott, D. W. (1947) *Hate in the countertransference in collected papers: through paediatrics to psychoanalysis*. London, Tavistock, pp. 194–203

Winnicott, D. W. (1953) Transitional objects and transitional phenomena: a study of the first not-me possession. *International Journal of Psychoanalysis*. 34, 89–97.

Chapter 3

Considering perversion from a Portman Clinic perspective[1]

Donald Campbell

Introduction

Psychoanalysis has always been to a greater or lesser extent politically incorrect. Psychoanalytic thinking about perversion has aroused condemnation from the right of the intellectual and political spectrum, and criticism that we have got it all wrong from gay rights activists and feminist writers. Two quotes from Freud are particularly relevant. The first comes from his paper on *A Case of Hysteria* that was written, for the most part, in January 1901:

> All psycho-neurotics are persons with strongly marked perverse tendencies, which had been repressed in the course of their development and had become unconscious. Consequently their unconscious *phantasies* show precisely the same content as the documentarily recorded *actions* of perverts .... Psycho-neuroses are, so to speak, *negative* perversions. In neurotics the sexual constitution, under which the effects of heredity are included, operate in combination with any accidental influences in their life, which may disturb the development of normal sexuality. A stream of water which meets with an obstacle in the river-bed is damned up and flows back into old channels which had formerly seemed fated to run dry. (pp. 50–51)

Freud reminds us that none of us can stand in a superior judgemental position in relation to those who suffer from perversions. I assume that all of us in one way or another are neurotic and have entertained perverse fantasies. If Freud is right, all of us have within us a resource in our unconscious fantasies to understand the use we make of sexual fantasies and behaviour, including perverse behaviour.

Returning to the theme of psychoanalysis as politically incorrect, so many of Freud's discoveries have become an acceptable part of the fabric of our culture that you might be surprised to know that if you had wanted to hear Freud give the lectures that were to become the *Three Essays on the Theory of Sexuality* in 1905, you would have had to cross a picket line because people were outraged at the thought that children had a sex life.

In this chapter, I will address the subject of sadism because the desire to inflict pain upon the sexual object and to have it inflicted upon oneself is, as Freud (1905) maintained in the *Three Essays*, '...the most common and the most significant of all the perversions...' (p. 157). I will focus particularly on sadism as a solution to primitive anxieties about survival.

The self-preservative function of the ego

Freud viewed the ego's primary function to be the preservation of the self. We share this primary aim with all living creatures. A constitutional predisposition to preserve the species underpins the individual's protective and reproductive behaviour. We can see graphic illustrations of fight/flight mechanisms on wildlife documentaries. Sometimes our excitement and tension in the stalking and the fight, our revulsion in the killing, our fear and awe of the predator, or our sympathy for the victim make it difficult to remember that animals compete for territory and mates and kill for food in order to survive. We are witnessing self-preservative aggression.

Human beings experience threats to survival from far more complex sources than food, shelter and sexual reproduction. Sometimes, attacks on vulnerable children, or the ill or elderly, or the sheer scale of violence, such as the horrific events in New York City and Washington on 9/11 generate such rage, pain and grief that is difficult to think about the perpetrator's motivation. It may be difficult to understand the attacks on the World Trade Centre and the Pentagon as dramatic examples of aggression in response to a perceived threat to survival. At a conscious level, terrorists are fighting for the survival of their ideology, which they believe is threatened by the domination of Judaeo-Christian and capitalist belief systems. The religious beliefs of the terrorists give them a psychic cohesiveness: they define who they are, and give meaning to their lives and, most importantly, to their deaths. This kind of internal world, supported by faith in a reward of eternal life, makes this type of aggression the most dangerous to combat. Viewed from this perspective, the self-preservative nature of the terrorist's violence becomes clearer, but no less horrific or excusable.

I have begun with recent and graphic illustrations of violence, which is motivated by a self-preservative instinct, to illustrate its destructiveness and the complex nature of the psychological ingredients that humans depend upon for their survival. While the mix of beliefs and internal objects is always idiosyncratic, each of us is motivated to maintain a psychic steady state or homeostatic balance between the internal and external world. The ego's task is to negotiate compromise where there is conflict between the inside and outside in order to achieve stability and balance. The ego organizes conscious and unconscious fantasies as solutions to competing and fluctuating internal and external demands, which threaten the homeostasis of the internal world (Sandler & Sandler, 1992).

Therefore, the 'best' solution negotiated by the ego is that which creates and maintains a feeling of safety and well-being. A neurotic or psychotic state, a symptom, or a character trait, a defence mechanism or a perversion, however maladapted in the outside world, may be the 'best' solution the ego can negotiate given the external circumstances and the ego's internal resources (Sandler & Sandler, 1992), which, in turn, are built upon constitutional and environmental factors. Sexuality and aggression, with their accompanying fantasies and enactments, are our most fundamental resources for the resolution of our problems.

In psychoanalysis we can see that current fantasies, developed as solutions to conflicts in the present, were permeated to a greater or lesser extent by primitive fantasies representing solutions to earlier developmental conflicts. For instance, paranoid fantasies in response to no real threat are likely to be based on earlier solutions to anxieties about safety. These archaic fantasies define our character, aims and behaviour.

Ruthless aggression

I would now like to turn to the subject of earlier developmental conflicts, particularly those that arouse anxieties about survival, and sketch out for you a model for the development of sadism, its role and function. Later I will illustrate these issues with some clinical material.

When I view the ego's primary function as the preservation of the self, I am referring to anything that constitutes a threat to physical or psychological homeostasis. This includes, in this context, narcissistic equilibrium, that is the maintenance of a dynamic balance, a steady state at optimum levels. Bio-physiologists such as Cannon (1939) have shown that the body has an elaborate reflexive reaction pattern that prepares it for fight or flight in the presence of danger, ideas taken forward in contemporary understandings of trauma and the autonomic nervous system (Porges, 2011).

In the psychic sphere, ruthless aggression is triggered as a fundamental, immediate and substantial response to any threat to the self with the aim of negating this source of danger. All of us as infants and adults are capable of ruthless aggression.

I am using the term violence to refer to a physical response of aggression while the term aggression I use to denote a psychical response. Ruthless aggression, whether expressed physically or psychically, has a single aim of getting rid of a threat and the relation to the object is not relevant once the threat has been eliminated.

If you suddenly found yourself being stalked by a lion in the African bush and unable to run, you would normally react with self-preservative aggression with the aim of getting rid of the lion. A distinguishing feature of ruthless aggression is it's single-minded, narrow-vision quality like a laser beam, which focuses on the dangerousness of the object rather than the object itself. If the victim's look is experienced as threatening through accusation, it is the eyes that are attacked; if what is being said is intolerable, the mouth is punched, and so on (Glasser, 1998: p. 888). In infants or extreme situations, the laser beam quality is lost and violence is directed indiscriminately.

You may be thinking that there are certain forms of violence that are self-preservative but do not appear to be aimed at negating a danger such as 'predatory violence' (Meloy, 1988: p. 25). When we thought about the lion from the prey's point of view, as the lion was stalking us, we could think of the lion's threat as an example of predatory violence. However, when we look at the dynamics of the attack from the lion's point of view, we can see that the lion is motivated not by the prey's edibility, but rather by the danger of its unavailability, the risk of the prey escaping. As Lantos recognizes: 'the animal hunting its prey is driven by hunger. Hunger makes it angry, but his anger is not directed against the prey. On the contrary he is pleased when it comes his way. No subjective aggression is felt while chasing, catching, tearing, biting and swallowing it' (1958: p. 118).

During a moment of ruthless aggression or violence the object holds no personal significance other than his/her dangerousness: it is carried out in the interest of self-preservation and any other considerations have no relevance. The response of the object in any other respect is of no interest (Glasser, 1998: p. 891).

With this view of the nature and function of ruthless aggression in mind, I turn now to the mother and her infant. Threats to the infant's psyche and/or physical survival (the infant cannot not be expected to know the difference between them) normally mobilize ruthless aggression directed towards the object, which is perceived as dangerous. The threat may be experienced as a direct assault, engulfment, smothering or abandonment to starve. As I had explained earlier the aim of self-preservative aggression is to negate the threat.

However, when the object that is perceived as threatening to the child's survival is the same object upon which it depends for its survival – the mother – the exercise of ruthless aggression poses a dilemma for the child. How can the infant survive the unmitigated and unmediated terror of the other? How is the child to survive if it cannot afford to get rid of mother? How can it survive the consequences of its omnipotent violence? Children tend to fashion an ingenious solution by libidinizing their aggression towards the mother, that is fusing love for mother with aggression towards her. In this way the child changes the aim of aggression from eliminating mother to controlling her in a libidinally gratifying way. Ruthless aggression is, thereby, converted into sadism. The ego now has two types of aggression with which to pursue it's aim of protecting the self against any threat to it's survival: ruthless aggression and sadist aggression.

The role of sadism

In a ruthless response where the aim is, by fight or flight, to eliminate the threat to one's survival, the impact upon the object is irrelevant beyond the achievement of this aim. However, in a sadistic attack, the relationship to the object must be preserved, not eliminated. By radically altering the relationship to the threatening object to ensure that both self and object survive, sadism now offers the child a second line of defence.

Subtly modulated mild sadomasochism emerges now as a libidinal component of the good enough bond between mother and child. However, when the mother's sadism is not tempered by reparation or extends beyond the child's capacity to recover a nurturing image, or when mother's narcissism makes it impossible for her to be aware of her infant's needs and respond appropriately, the child may rely on more frequent and more intense sadomasochistic exchanges to control a not good enough mother.

I observed an interaction between an infant and its mother which illustrated the shift from ruthless aggression to sadism. As an analytic student, I observed on a weekly basis a mother feeding her infant. I noticed that the mother often teased the baby by pulling her nipple away from her sucking child and moving it just out of reach as the child groped with its mouth to find and latch on to the nipple again. The mother laughed as she did this while her child became frustrated, tense and eventually enraged. On several occasions, the child collapsed into cries. It was painful to watch. After watching this for about six weeks, I noticed that the child did not respond by pursuing the nipple or becoming tense and angry. Instead, the child stopped, looked up at the mother and smiled. The mother then returned the nipple to her child's mouth. I thought that smile represented a libidinization of the aggression that had previously been mobilized by the frustration the child experienced in the pursuit of the withdrawn nipple. With its feed and survival at stake the child appeared to identify with the mother's sadism to respond to the mother sadistically and, as a result, regain control the unavailable breast.

The core complex

Glasser (1979, 1992) has identified a complex which he refers to as the *core complex* because it occurs universally in normal development and begins with the infant's wish to merge with an idealized, omnipotently gratifying mother as an early solution to anxieties of loss engendered by its own moves towards separation and individuation (see Mahler, Pine & Bergman, 1975). We can observe these conflicts quite graphically during the separation and individuation phase of development, but they occur throughout the life cycle. The success of the merging 'solution' depends upon: (1) a good enough mother who is able to respond to her child's needs at the right time with enough comfort, protection and nourishment and (2) a good enough father who can protect the child from mother's failures and provide an alternative to the exclusive fused relationship with her.

However, the child with a weak and or unavailable father is vulnerable if mother is narcissistically oriented. A narcissistic mother responds to her child on the basis of her own needs, giving too much too soon, or not enough when it is too late. The child may experience this type of mother as engulfing, intruding or smothering, on the one hand, or indifferent, abandoning and unreachable on the other. In either case, the child becomes acutely anxious about its survival. The infant that I observed was, I think, primarily anxious about abandonment and being left to starve. Such primitive anxieties about being able to find the object during the oral phase of development heighten anxieties later as the child moves towards separation and individuation.

This crisis in the *core complex* usually reaches a climax during the child's anal phase when it is preoccupied with urinary and faecal productions, and conflicts within itself and its parents over control of these pleasurable functions and admirable creations. It is not surprising that a child might borrow from its solutions to conflicts over control of its body to fashion ingenious but maladaptive solutions which enable him or her to retain his or her mother (after a fashion) and to survive (at a price). In this way crisis in development around proximity to the object, that is anxieties about engulfment on the one hand and abandonment on the other, become negotiated through sadism which then becomes a solution to anxieties about the revival of these earlier conflicts in later phases of development. Later I will refer to clinical material, which, I hope, will illustrate the anxieties associated with the *core complex*.

The development of a perversion

The vicissitudes of the sadomasochistic interaction between the mother, her child, and the father influence the nature of the conflicts against which a perversion defends. When the mother's sadism fails to defend her against what she experiences as her child's persecution, she may be at risk of abandoning her sadistic treatment of her child and rely upon ruthless aggression or it psychic equivalent. The child's well-being is then no longer relevant to the mother. Her only concern is negating or eliminating any aspect of the child that poses *a threat to her survival*. At this point the child's development, or, indeed, it's life, is at greatest risk.

Initially the child responds to what is experienced as an accelerating risk to its survival by intensifying its sadistic control of an increasingly dangerous object, such as a borderline or psychotic mother, and the threat of breakdown. But what recourse does the child have if it's sadism fails to satisfactorily control a psychotic mother? In such cases, the child is likely to abandon it's sadomasochistic relationship with the object and, like its mother, regress to reliance upon ruthless aggression with the aim of eliminating a too-painful reality by psychotic withdrawal or destruction of it's internal objects.

When the line of development from ruthless aggression to the libidinization of aggression progresses to the intensification of sadism, the psychic groundwork is laid for the development of perverse solutions to neurotic or psychotic conflicts. By extending this line of development to where intensified sadism becomes the dominating organizer of libidinal life, we reach the point where perversions become structured.

The aim of defence in the perversions (Glover, 1933, 1956) is to preserve enough reality sense to be able to function, even in a limited way, in the real world. By reducing paranoid dangers, by whatever means, the individual 'gains breathing space' to assess objective reality. However, the cost of this adaptation is the sacrifice of that part of reality, which threatens the individual's survival. A perversion may defend against the dangers represented by psychotic anxieties from pre-Oedipal sources, such as internal chaos, fragmentation or disintegration of the ego; or against the neurotic anxieties arising out of unresolved Oedipal conflicts, such as castration, infantile sexuality, or narcissistic wounds. Whatever the source of the danger, the individual's orientation to reality will be affected.

Rycroft suggests that someone who is on the border between neurosis and psychosis either defies categorization, or is someone whose mechanisms are psychotic but whose behaviour does not warrant his being treated as psychotic. 'The usage arises from the fact that diagnostic systems assume that neurosis and psychosis are mutually exclusive, which clinical observation show they are not' (1968: p. 14). Given the ambiguity of the term, it could still be argued that one of the differences between the perverse solution in the hysteric and the perverse solution in the borderline person is the amount of reality that the perversion has preserved. The perverse solution in the borderline individual preserves less reality than it does in the neurotic.

Chasseguet-Smirgel (1985) points out that the 'bedrock of reality is created by the difference between the sexes and the difference between generations: the inevitable period of time separating a child from his mother (for whom he is an inadequate sexual partner) and from his father (whose potent adult sexual organ he does not possess) .... The perverse temptation leads one to accept pregenital desire and satisfactions (attainable by the small boy) as being equal to or even superior to genital desires and satisfactions (attainable only by the father). Erosion of the double difference between the sexes and the generations is the pervert's objective' (p. 2). This dynamic lies behind the perverse patient's attacks on thinking and linking because of the dangers arising out of the internal and external reality of intercourse. Consequently, the dangers against which the perversion defends will inevitability affect the subject's relationship with the object's sexuality and, for the paedophile, its relationship with the generation of children and adolescents.

I will refer to some clinical material from the case of Mr J in order to illustrate the defensive function of sadistic perversion, with special reference to fantasy.

The case of Mr. J

Mr. J was a handsome dark-haired 21 year old with a self-conscious extravert manner. He made a special point of telling me in our first interview that he was actively heterosexual and has had several girlfriends.

Mr. J's father was a probation officer whom he respected and loved. He regarded his father as clever, easy-going, friendly and caring, but not emotionally close during his childhood and adolescence. Mother was seen as an hysterical extravert who was not really interested in him. I learned that before his parents divorced, his mother had been fascinated by gay clubs and had taken her husband to them.

Mr. J saw himself as obedient and pliable until his parents divorced when he was 12 and father left him at home with his mother who treated him like a 'kicking post'. He began truanting and was obnoxious and defiant towards older men and male teachers. However, he was impressed by the flamboyance of the gay nightclub scene, and after leaving school he worked in gay clubs serving customers while wearing a pair of shorts with braces. It was there that he met a wealthy Greek man and eventually moved in with him.

Mr. J recalled the night he and his homosexual lover took his mother to a gay club. He particularly remembers his mother smiling with approval when he and his lover held hands. Eventually, Mr. J acknowledged his bitter disappointment that his mother had abandoned his heterosexual development and was excited by his homosexual attachment.

Two months later, he moved out after meeting a new girlfriend. Mr. J became sexually promiscuous with women and had no respect for them, but felt that he had to prove himself as a man, often comparing himself in a negative way with his current girlfriend's ex-boyfriend. Still later, Mr. J told me with embarrassment about his first homosexual relationship when he was 18 with an older flat mate with whom he indulged in mutual masturbation. He asked his friend to urinate on him and the friend agreed.

Mr. J recalled that it was at about the time of his parents' separation that he became aroused by young girls. He eventually told me that he masturbated to fantasies of eight-year-old girls. This emerged when Jane, his current girlfriend, had an abortion. The abortion stimulated anxieties about intimacy and fears of being annihilated by women, which he defended against through sadistic fantasies involving young girls and 'jamming my cock into their mouths'. He felt strong as he wrapped his arms around their pure clean bodies. He consciously thought of 6-year-olds as adults and had no sense of the generational boundaries or bodily barriers. Mr. J thought about children all the time. With shame and guilt, he told me that he would spend his spare time hunting young girls in council flats. Pre-pubertal girls found his charm irresistible. He regularly exposed his genitals to young girls in the street and invited others up to his flat on a pretext of playing an exciting game and then touched their genitals.

It emerged that Mr. J's fantasy about young girls included mothers who procured daughters for him, wittingly or unwittingly making their children available directly or by failing to keep them safe. He recounted his exploits with little girls to demonstrate my inability to stop him, as his father had failed to stake a claim for his son and provide an alternative to his seductive mother. In the transference it became clear that Mr. J wanted to elicit a gratifying collusion with me, his mother in the transference, that is someone who would be voyeuristically excited by his sadistic use of children. At a deeper level, Mr. J had projected the despair and confusion he felt with his mother onto little girls, seduced them into dependence upon him and then shocked them with a moment of betrayal when he touched their genitals.

Near the end of his therapy, Mr. J told me that he brought a kitten back to his room, even though his flat mate had told him from the beginning that animals were not allowed in the flat. Mr. J then told me that he planned to take the kitten to his mother to see if she would look after it for him. The cat represented Mr. J's inability to think realistically about caring for another object. However, this incident was also understood as an enactment of Mr. J's experience of himself as the lost kitten, which he could not look after, and his wish for his mother to properly care for him.

Unfortunately, Mr. J's recognition of an uncared for, unwanted kitten-self became intolerable for him and uncontainable in his therapy. He reversed the experience of being left by his father by abruptly terminating his treatment after a year. In this way, he also protected his illusion of adult heterosexuality in the face of unacceptable homosexual wishes, which were revived in the transference as he began to trust me more.

Mr. J's experience of being his mother's 'kicking post' mobilized ruthless aggression, which was libidinized, that is transformed into sadism, and directed towards little girls who did not pose the same threat as his mother or girlfriend. In this way Mr. J utilized paedophilia to preserve his objects and insure his survival.

Homosexuality

Psychoanalysis has been unfairly criticized for seeing homosexuality as a perversion in the same way fetishism, paedophilia, etc. In the case of Mr J, we can see that his anxiety about his homosexuality led to a flight into heterosexuality promiscuity, which reflected his anxieties about intimacy with women. This contributed to his retreat into sadistic fantasies of sex with young girls, who would be unable to threaten or resist him. He then acted upon those fantasies by touching the girls' genitals.

Freud (1920) distinguished between homosexuality and other sexual aberrations, arguing that homosexuals who come into treatment are not representative of the whole group; many homosexuals are not ill, cannot be 'cured', and can relate to others as whole objects, and there is a capacity for love, concern and sublimation. The homosexuals whom I have seen at the Portman Clinic are not typical of the group as a whole; they are violent and perverse, and their sexuality is disturbing either to themselves or other people. The subject is contentious. It is probably more accurate to speak of different kinds of homosexuality, as one would refer to types of hetero-sexuality, but that would lead us into another paper. Nor is sexual or-ientation necessarily fixed; Mr. J, for example, can be seen to be retreating from homosexuality into a fascination with young girls, and many people are actively bisexual, or find their sexual orientation changes over time.

Aggression as reactive or instinctual

A view that perversion arises out of the vicissitudes of aggression takes the reader into an area of psychoanalytic theory where there is widespread disagreement. This chapter can do no more than briefly sketch some of the contending theories about the nature of aggression.

Self-preservative aggression has been described in this chapter as a primal reaction pattern triggered by danger. However, many psychoanalysts follow Freud, who viewed aggression as a drive with its need for discharge of or-ganically based energy. Freud's instinct theory has never been substantiated (see Glasser, 1998; Hartmann et al., 1949), and is currently under scrutiny from believers and non-believers alike. For instance, Feldman (2000), an advocate of the death drive, uses a case study to argue that the aim of the death instinct is not to kill or annihilate the object, but to maintain a link with the object, albeit a tormenting one. According to Michael Feldman, gratification is not derived from a fusion with the life instinct and con-sequent libidinization, but is 'an essential element of such a destructive drive' (p. 64).

James Grotstein (2000) thinks that viewing the death drive as antagonistic to the life instinct is misleading. He views the death instinct as another di-mension of the life instinct with a protective and adaptive function that allows for 'partial-to-total death of the mind if the mothering person fails to attune, hold, and/or contain her infant's inchoate infinite distress' (p. 477).

At the other end of the psychoanalytic spectrum, David Black (2001), following his analysis of Freud's arguments based on evolution and neuroa-natomy in support of his hypothesis of a death drive, concludes that the death instinct was a detour of historical interest to psychoanalysis, but, 'as such, probably merits no future in psychoanalytic thinking' (p. 185). However, paradoxically, the death drive proved to be fruitful for future developments in psychoanalysis. Black draws attention to Freud's notion of the mutual 'binding' of the drives that is particularly germane to my emphasis in this paper on the libidinization of aggression, which transforms gratification that results from aggressive negation of the object to gratification being derived from control of the object. In this way, self-preservative aggression becomes sadism.

Some thoughts about working with individuals who suffer from a perversion

Translating an understanding of perversion into an effective treatment is an extremely difficult and complex process. Psychoanalysis as a treatment discipline relies upon the recognition and understanding of the transference, that is the transfer of wishes, fantasies and anxieties associated with important people from one's past onto the analyst, and the counter transference, which is the analyst's pre-conscious or unconscious reaction to the impact of the transference. There are two aspects of the transference which are played out in a session; (1) the patient's perception of the analyst as a transference figure and (2) the patient's evocation or provocation of the analyst in order to actualize elements of the transference, that is to bring to life in the session the object the patient expects to find. The transference functions as a resistance to psychotherapy and to the recognition and working through of anxieties derived from early conflicts and traumas

Consequently, the analytic clinician would expect the perverse patient to relate to the therapist with the same defences as those he employs in his or her perversion. When we return to Mr J, the patient in the case example, we can see that he relied upon projection to control unbearable aspects of his inner world by assaulting young girls. Mr J, who was adept at relating to little girls at their level in order to win their confidence, trust and hope, was preoccupied with trying to win my trust and inspire hope in the effectiveness of therapy. Patients, like Mr J, will be skilled at 'reading' the practitioner's valuation of his own work and can readily 'co-operate' with assessment or therapy, or simulate attitudes and behaviours consciously or unconsciously promoted by caretakers. The individual suffering from a sexual deviation is likely to rely upon compliance, imitation and simulation to protect himself from the intrusion and rejection he expects from the authority figures represented by the diagnostician, therapist or any professional, just as he did with his parents.

Those working with people suffering from a perversion will be familiar with this phenomenon. This is not a self-conscious pretence. Just as the paedophile actually believes that he or she is their child victim's best friend, sensitive babysitter or helpful tutor, he or she actually believes they are good clients who are co-operating by acknowledging their abusive behaviour, etc.

These simulations are believable for the professional because the perpetrator is a believer himself (Campbell, 1994).

Nevertheless, the true self beneath the compliance will wage a 'guerrilla campaign' against the therapeutic process that, he believes, aims to take him over completely, just as his abuser had. The subtle or gross signs of resistance offer the professional a more reliable clue to the whereabouts of the true self which may be so deeply buried that even the patient has lost contact with it. It is unlikely that the seriously disturbed sexually deviant person will ever find his or her way back to their actual self without the help of a professional.

However, any individual or group treatment or management programme that adopts a macho or an authoritarian role, or focuses exclusively on behavioural change without understanding the individual's internal conflicts and anxieties is in danger of being sabotaged by the abuser's capacity to adopt language, concepts and whatever is suggested as normative behaviour, in the same way as the chameleon takes on the colour of its environment as a protection against attack. Since the change is based on simulated attitudes and behaviour, it only *appears* to be change. Momentarily, one will see changes in the abuser's behaviour as the result of this kind of identification with the therapist, probation officer, child care protection worker, etc., but, since underlying anxieties are not affected, the abuser is at risk of returning to abusive behaviour once the external supports have been taken away and old anxieties re-emerge. Put into the language of child abuse, any treatment or management programme that does not take the abuser's internal world into account is very likely to be victimized by the abuser in the same way as the child victims are, that is by being deceived by the outwardly positive but inwardly fraudulent behaviour of these clients. When professionals discover they have been deceived they should guard against reacting in an abusive way by abandoning their clients or adopting a punitive attitude (Campbell, 1994).

Conclusion

Moralizing and 'political correctness' have interfered with efforts to understand the perplexing subject of perversion. There is no place for moral judgements and politics in the psychoanalytic study and treatment of perversion. Freud reminds us that we all have within us the roots of perverse development. Perversions occur in both sexes, adults and adolescents, heterosexuals as well as homosexuals. From a psychoanalytic perspective, no one has the right to cast the first stone.

The task of translating an understanding of perversion into effective treatment is extremely difficult and complex. The practitioner will be hampered by the limited state of knowledge of perversion, and by his own unconscious processes and unresolved conflicts. In order to be effective, mental health practitioners and psychoanalysts have to continually scrutinize themselves for prejudice, fears, phobias or anxieties associated with perverse fantasies or behaviour. Any psychoanalytically oriented treatment is an intersubjective process involving not only the professional but also the perverse individual who may play a role in his subsequent abuse within the treatment. For instance, a person suffering from a perversion may expect the therapist or social worker or 'the system' to relate to him in an abusive way, based on his experience of the way his mother and father related to him. It is not unusual for such a patient to attempt to provoke the professional into a response of punishment or collusion (such as feeling sorry for an abuser in such a way as to avoid recognition and understanding of his or her maliciousness), in order to confirm the patient's expectation that he won't be taken seriously as a whole person.

Note

1 This chapter is a revised version of an earlier paper (Campbell, 2005).

References

Black, D. (2001) Mapping a detour: why did Freud speak of a death drive? *British Journal of Psychotherapy.* 18 (2), 185–198.

Campbell, D. (1994) Breaching the shame shield: thoughts on the assessment of adolescent child sexual abusers. *Journal of Child Psychotherapy.* 20, 309–326.

Campbell, D. (2005) Perversion: sadism and survival. In: Budd, S. & Rushbridger, R. (eds.) *Introducing psychoanalysis.* London, Routledge. pp. 231–245.

Cannon, W. B. (1939) *The wisdom of the body.* London, Kegan Paul, Trench, Trubner.

Chasseguet-Smirgel, J. (1985) *Creativity and perversion.* London, Free Association Books.

Feldman, M. (2000) Some views on the manifestation of the death instinct in clinical work. *The International Journal of Psychoanalysis.* 81, 53–65.

Freud, S. (1901) A case of hysteria, *SE.* VII, 1–309.

Freud, S. (1905) Three essays on the theory of sexuality, *SE.* VII, 136–248.

Freud, S. (1920) Beyond the pleasure principle. *SE.* XVIII, 3–64.

Glasser, M. (1979) Some aspects of the role of aggression in the perversions. In: Rosen, I. (ed.) *Sexual deviations.* 2nd ed. Oxford, Oxford University Press. pp. 278–305.

Glasser, M. (1992) Problems in the psychoanalysis of certain narcissistic disorders. *The International Journal of Psychoanalysis.* 73, 493–503.

Glasser, M. (1998) On violence – a preliminary communication. *The International Journal of Psychoanalysis.* 79, 887–902.

Glover, E. (1933) The relation of perversion-formation to the development of reality sense. *The International Journal of Psychoanalysis.* 14, 4. (This paper also appears in: Glover, E. (1956) *On the early development of the mind,* London, Imago, 13, pp. 216–234.)

Grotstein, J. (2000) Some considerations of "hate" and a reconsideration of the death instinct. *Psychoanalytic Inquiry.* 20, 462–480.

Hartmann, H. et al. (1949) Notes on the theory of aggression. *The Psychoanalytic Study of the Child.* 3, 9–36.

Lantos, B. (1958) The two genetic derivations of aggression with reference to sublimation and neutralisation. *The International Journal of Psychoanalysis.* 39, 116–120.

Mahler, M., Pine, F., & Bergman, A. (1975) *The psychological birth of the human infant.* London, Hutchinson & Co Ltd.

Meloy, J. R. (1988) *The psychopathic mind – origins, dynamics and treatment.* London, Jason Aronson.

Porges, S. W. (2011) *The polyvagal theory: neurophysiological foundations of emotions, attachment, communication, and self-regulation.* New York, Norton.

Rycroft, C. (1968) *A critical dictionary of psychoanalysis.* London, Nelson.

Sandler, J. & Sandler, A.-M. (1992) Psychoanalytic technique and theory of psychic change. *Bulletin Anna Freud Centre.* 15, 35–51.

Chapter 4

Young people in difficulty with internet sex and pornography

Graham Music and Heather Wood

Digital worlds, online sexual stimuli and new challenges

The internet and digital technology confront us with new challenges. Increasing numbers of young people are presenting with compulsive use of internet sex and pornography, alongside other compulsive internet use. This chapter describes some of the ways in which engagement with internet sex can impact on young people's sexual development and become problematic and some of the clinical challenges of working with these issues. In this developing area of work, we are inevitably still exploring how best to approach these problems.

A 2017 study (Hamilton-Giachritis et al., 2017) commissioned by NSPCC and the Children's Commissioner suggested that 65% of mid-adolescent boys had seen pornography online, and most thought such images were realistic. Thirty-six per cent had taken sexually explicit 'selfies' and been asked to share these online. These figures are probably conservative. The report also described a process of habituation, in which initial exposure could give rise to a degree of shock at what was being viewed, which quickly waned.

Young men seen at the Portman Clinic who present with a problematic relationship to internet sex, tend to be in their late teens or early 20s; the girls and young women who are seen are more likely to be involved in sexting or making themselves vulnerable to online victimization, and tend to be younger, with the majority in their early teens. Most are seen for once-weekly therapy. In England and Wales, pornography is deemed illegal if it depicts people under the age of 18. Some of the young people seen will have Social Services' involvement if they are themselves vulnerable, or there may be Youth Offending or Probation involvement if they have been found guilty of possession or distribution of illegal images. As with all therapeutic work at the Portman Clinic, each patient will have a Case Manager who liaises with external agencies if necessary, to enable to therapist to work with the patient in a boundaried way.

Themes and challenges of the work

Adolescence is a crucial period of psychosexual development. Among the many tasks of adolescence, the young person needs to assimilate into their sense of themselves their new-found sexual body with adult sexual characteristics, indeed, Laufer (1976) argues that this is the main developmental task of adolescence, under which other 'tasks' are subsumed. The young person needs to make a shift from being the child of a sexual couple, to seeing themselves as a sexual adult capable of making a couple of their own. If incestuous relations are to be avoided, this involves a shift from having a primary investment in familial relationships, to having a primary investment in extra-familial relationships. It also involves a shift from sexual activities focused exclusively on the self (masturbatory/auto-erotic), to activities also involving a partner, and the development of a capacity to manage all that this entails, including exposure of the physical body, acceptance of another's body, tolerance of intimacy and tolerance of ambivalence. The establishment of an adult sexual identity also entails finding forms of sexual expression that reflect, not only the gender identity and sexual orientation of the individual but also the expression of dominant patterns of relating in intimate relationships. One person will seek to be cared for in intimate relationships, while another will seek to excite or arouse and a third person may feel compelled to dominate the other. These underlying object relationships will shape sexual as well as non-sexual behaviours.

The developmental processes specific to adolescence are complex and subject to disruption by adverse experiences. A very significant proportion of young people learn about sex from the internet, and it can be a valuable source of information and education, but internet use also has the power to disrupt psychological defences, engendering excitement and omnipotence, encouraging narcissistic and part-object forms of relating, appearing to condone the sadistic treatment of the online 'other' and undermining superego functioning (see Wood, 2011). When these more general aspects of internet use are coupled with exposure to vast amounts of uncensored and extreme sexual imagery, this can significantly impact on a young person's sexual development. Internet pornography frequently offers distorted or exaggerated images of the adult sexual body; idealized, dehumanized or sadistic versions of sexual engagement and easy access to imagery of sexual 'mothers', 'fathers' and children, thus trampling all over what might be fragile Oedipal or generational sexual boundaries. Young people and adults describe how sexual imagery to which they are exposed during this formative period can become etched in their minds, hard to forget or transcend. The individual is invited to participate in sexual scenarios through fantasy and masturbation, creating an imaginary world where they can distance themselves from a troubled experience of their changing body. Lemma (2014) describes how '*cyberspace is ideally suited to being defensively used to bypass the psychic implications of an embodied self* (p.78). As often happens, it is those who are already more emotionally vulnerable who will be most at risk.

Our experience of working with adults and young people who are compulsively using internet pornography or engaging in internet sex, is that, although they may spend a considerable amount of time sexually aroused, actually they are often very disconnected from their own bodily experiences and desires. It is not uncommon for people to become reliant on the external stimulation of the provided image, but to be unable to become aroused through internally-generated sexual fantasy. In some people, the use of internet pornography seems to be used defensively in order 'not to know about' internally-generated desires. We have particularly observed this where there are cultural and religious prohibitions on sexuality. In this respect, these problems can bear some resemblance to accounts of hysteria. Bollas (2000) describes how *'the hysteric seeks to remain a sexual innocent whilst relieving itself (sic) of its excitations in fantasy. Auto-erotic sexuality seems permissible, even if the content of the fantasies suggests sexual relations to the other. Auto-erotic sexuality is private, tucked away, hidden from the other'* (p.164).

In the consulting room, the experience of being with these patients, who describe a surfeit of sexual excitement and activity, is often of feeling rather flat and dead. The work can feel boring. It is as though, underneath this excess of excitement and arousal, there is a sense of something depressed, or deathly, or disconnected. The work of therapy may then be to find the life in the individual, the spontaneous feeling or desire, and to understand why this is under attack or cannot be tolerated, leading to it becoming hijacked or replaced by this 'virtual' version of sexual expression.

Immersion in internet sex can provide a refuge, not just from anxieties about the body and sexuality, but from the challenges of intimate relationships. For the young person, entry into the world of sexual relationships can seem a perilous journey. Will they desire and be desired, will intimacy be experienced as abusive or intrusive, will it stir up primitive longings for merger and fusion?

A concept central to our work at the Portman Clinic is the notion of the core complex, proposed by Mervyn Glasser in 1979. Glasser's core complex describes the longing for blissful fusion with another – the wish to merge with another and lose oneself in an in-love state of union. But to merge with another threatens loss of self and potential annihilation and evokes aggression towards the other who might take us over in this way, but who is the very object of desire. There are different solutions to this – one solution is narcissistic withdrawal, where we give up trying to engage with the other and retreat to a state of isolation but feel depressed and lonely. Glasser proposes that the solution found by people who go on to develop perversions is that they stay engaged with the other, but treat them sadistically, where the sadism is a vehicle for the expression of the aggression stirred up by the desirable object. Here the object is not destroyed by the aggression, but is treated cruelly and made to suffer. The core complex is a kind of claustro-agoraphobic dilemma: to be close threatens claustrophobia, but to be alone threatens unbearable loneliness. For one young man, Saul, it was the transition from being with another to being alone which was tortuous. He often turned to pornography after an enjoyable evening out with friends, as if the transition from connection to solitude was unbearable and had to be bridged by the fantasy of intimacy with another. Pornography became a way of protecting himself from the ambivalence and fear of engagement, and from knowing about absence and loss. Towards the end of the therapy, he spoke of how masturbating with pornography felt like having someone else there – or the closest he could allow himself to get to having someone else there. Looking, admiring, being turned on by appearances may be an inevitable part of sex. But in this situation, an excited looking substitutes for the challenges of being with another in an emotional and a bodily way.

Therapeutic work, while not involving bodily contact or exposure, can confront the young person with just those aspects of intimacy which they fear – exposure of their vulnerability, the risk of stirring up powerful feelings of conflict and ambivalence, and anxieties in relation to the other of being taken over, or abused, or rejected. Often the patient's fears are defended against by making the therapist feel 'small', unexciting, and of no interest compared to the auto-erotic pleasures of the internet. What does therapy have to offer when compared with limitless images of sexual scenarios? In the countertransference one often has to tolerate being made to feel either very boring, or powerless, when compared with the enticements of internet sex.

The compulsive use of internet sex can therefore be like an excess of bodily arousal used to treat a disconnection from the 'embodied' self of sexuality and feeling; it can be like an excess of sexual excitement used to treat an absence of sexual desire, or used to mask highly conflicted sexual desire, or used to mask the terror of becoming emotionally and physically close to another.

The term 'sexualization' is used in psychoanalysis to denote, not straightforward sexual expression, but the use of sexuality as a defence, often a defence against core complex anxieties as Glasser described. Sexualization may be thought of as one of a group of manic defences. Sexual arousal is inherently exhilarating and energizing and lends itself to use as a manic defence. Aspects of physical arousal are confirmation that the body is alive and lively. In a state of arousal the person imagines themselves desired and desiring. Thus, this imparts powerful feelings of vitality and desire, and is a particularly convenient defence when the feelings to be countered are those of being depressed, deadened and undesirable. Once again this poses a challenge for the therapist. What we offer can be seen as very 'grey' and dull, essentially a life of 'depressive position' acceptance of ambivalence and imperfection, in contrast to the 'technicolour' world of endless sexual stimulation.

Compulsive use of internet sex is only a symptom, and as such, the underlying drivers can be many, varied and idiosyncratic. The case illustrations which follow are not intended to be comprehensive nor to represent best practice, but to offer a snapshot of the kind of issues that emerge in treatment. Because this is a highly sensitive area of work, case illustrations are from our own and others' practice, and are disguised or composites of a number of cases.

'Mano': using pornography to defend against painful feelings and a lack of body awareness

Mano, a late adolescent who moved to the UK with refugee parents at 8 years old, was struggling in school, and spending hours watching pornography alone in his room, reporting that he masturbated up to 18 times a day. The pornography that he watched was becoming increasingly violent, although still legal.

Both parents came from backgrounds of migration and ethnic discrimination. His parents were both regular church goers in an evangelical congregation. His mother had suffered much verbal abuse in her own childhood and his father had been quite absent in Mano's early years and, when present, used excessive physical chastisement. As a young boy Mano had ADHD-like symptoms, being fidgety, jumpy and unable to concentrate. He told of teachers tying one of his legs to a chair so he would stay sitting down.

He was a vigilant young man, alert to any noise outside the consulting room. Looking up at a window that had rattled, he noted, 'I know exactly what I would do if someone tried to climb through, I have planned how I would defend myself', explaining the martial arts moves he would enact. He noticed the tiniest changes in the room, such as a book being moved or something new on the desk.

While such compulsive pornography use and masturbation is increasingly common in young men, some, like Mano, have more proclivity for addictive behaviours. He often gorged on unhealthy food, and over-indulged in gaming. Mano's issues can be understood from many angles, but of relevance here was his inability to manage affect. It seemed he had never been helped to do so, and had had a lifelong struggle with emotional and bodily regulation.

The possibility for young people like Mano to retreat from painful experiences into more manic fantasies is facilitated by the internet. Waiting and delay are bypassed, and pornography and sexual excitement can serve as an immediate 'treatment' for any intolerable thought or feeling. It was quite some time before Mano could begin to make sense of the triggers that led him to seek such an escape, or even to recognize that he had had a difficult or painful feeling.

His mother reported high levels of anxiety while pregnant and in his early months. Probably Mano was born predisposed for stress, given how maternal stress affects the developing foetus (Music, 2016). Mother was depressed postnatally and reported that he was hard to soothe. She was not especially psychologically minded, probably limited in her ability to help him make sense of his experience in a containing and calming way.

In such environments, infants experience physiological signs of distress but do not have the experience of the bodily signal of distress being recognized, named and responded to by the caregiver, and in consequence, the arousal may feel overwhelming. Lacking the tools to recognize uncomfortable internal signals of arousal, distress or emotion, many children and adults learn to communicate and discharge feeling with their bodies, such as in sexual acting out or violence. Paradoxically they 'speak' with their bodies but are unaware of their body-states and the 'language' of emotions. Mano had poor interoceptive capacities, little ability to recognize emotions or body-states. Fonagy and Target (1998) describe the cluster of children who, in contrast to neurotic children, have poor capacity to mentalize, and often present at a very young age with intense, dramatic affect. By school age, like Mano, they may have attracted diagnoses of attention deficit hyperactivity disorder or conduct disorder as well as mood disorders, and by adolescence, *'drugs, food or promiscuous sex may be used to block feelings of being out of control, fragmented and lonely'* (p.91). 20 years on since the publication of this paper, compulsive use of internet sex and pornography is often observed in addition to these other presenting problems. In their view *'such patients need to learn to observe their own emotions and understand and label their emotional states, including their physiological and affective cues'* (p.105).

In such cases a classical psychoanalytic approach may need to be supplemented or preceded by an approach associated with Anna Freud (1978), known as 'developmental help', which recognizes that where there are developmental deficits it will be necessary to work with these first. In practice this may mean helping the patient to recognize and name bodily experiences and how these may be construed as feeling states, before being able to make use of an interpretive approach. Initially Mano's emotional vocabulary and range of known feeling states was minimal, mainly consisting of describing himself as 'cool' or 'good' (his positive affect states) or 'pissed' or 'shit' (his negative emotional range). There were few nuances to build on. Often, when I (GM) asked how he felt, he told me what he had been doing rather than describe a feeling. Trying to make sense of what had emotionally driven him to masturbatory acting-out was difficult.

He seemed to benefit from help with making basic links between his behaviours, impulses and their triggers. 'What has been happening?' I asked in one session several months in. Mano looked uneasy and then with something of a smirk told me that yesterday he 'wanked' nearly all afternoon. 'It's been bad' he said, but there was a notable discrepancy between his words and the emotions he communicated: I felt that he was pleased, triumphant and defiant, revelling in what Nathanson (2016) has described as pressing the 'fuck-it button', and communicating to me that he was in the grip of something way beyond my influence or control. In one session, at a noise of someone coming down the nearby stairs he jolted, looking around as if preparing for danger. I asked what was happening in his body in that moment, could he feel his heart beat, was it different to usual? He said, as often, 'I don't know'. I asked him to put his hand on his chest and feel his heart, which he did, almost to placate me, but became a little interested. It was of course beating quite fast. I suggested he keep his hand there and see if he could feel what happens in the next few minutes. He did and was surprised to note that he felt his heart-rate slow with his breath.

As Damasio (1999) observed, emotions are body-states which can be 'read', if we have the mental equipment with which to read them. With Mano, rather than interpret in a more formal way and offer my perception or construction of his experience, I tried to help him become aware of bodily signals of the emotional reactions he did not even know he had had. In a way that is typical of those caught up in compulsive sexual behaviours, initially he had no clue why he was masturbating so much, insisting he just 'liked it' or 'everyone needs a sexual outlet'. The complex meaning of sexual arousal or fantasy is stripped away, and we are to believe that this is just a biological necessity or expression of hedonism. Those few moments of pleasure when he ejaculated, he claimed, made life worthwhile. He craved this sensation like a drug addict craved their next hit.

This makes sense in terms of what we know about addictive processes. In all addictions, whether drugs, gambling, shopping, alcohol or pornography, the dopaminergic system is triggered. Key areas of such brain circuitry, such as the ventral striatum, are more activated at even the sight of a cue of their addiction, such as a laptop for a pornography user (Brand et al., 2016), or the bottle for the alcoholic (Kraus et al., 2016).

With pornography use we see habituation, people getting used to images which then become less stimulating, driving them to watch more exciting content, often violent or illegal. High pornography use in young men can also lead to sexual problems such as erectile dysfunction (Park et al., 2016). In addition pornography use seems implicated in lowering the capacity to delay gratification (Negash et al., 2016), and lessening activation of brain circuitry involved with empathy and executive functions.

Our dopaminergic system evolved for good reasons. It drives us towards what we need to survive and reproduce, such as sex and food. Yet this system can be hijacked by modern technology in a way that evolution has not prepared us for. Alluringly, technology offers the false hope of taking away feelings of sadness, anxiety or grief, promising respite from pain or difficulty.

Mano had been gloriously unaware of what triggered his addictions. It took a while before he became aware of signals from his body, such as the way his breathing changed when stressed. In time he became stiller, learning to be with and bear his feelings, to link his bodily states and emotions, and then link such emotions to his drives towards pornography or over-eating.

Interestingly, Mano spontaneously began to do yoga and mindfulness. In this period, he developed other capacities. For example, he started to read novels voraciously, itself a helpful thing, enhancing concentration, self-regulation and empathy (Kidd et al., 2016). These activities were all constructive but probably would have been insufficient without an experience of another mind that could attend to his experiences and recognize the ways in which his own mind could 'trick' him with promises of false solutions. In time he started to relinquish the pornography as he entered an intimate and fulfilling sexual relationship. He started to gravitate towards young people who were more emotionally literate, forming real friendships. In effect, he was developing the kind of capacities we see in secure attachment relationships. At the time of leaving therapy, he was in a stable relationship, had lost at least thirty pounds in weight, and reported that he had not masturbated compulsively for several months.

'Liam' : pornography as a 'solution' to the terrors of intimacy and as an electronic transitional object

Liam had grown up in a large family and his parents ran a family business, the relentless demands of which compounded his parents' reserved and unexpressive style of parenting. Liam said he felt loved, but there were no verbal statements of love, and it was only in therapy that he realized how lonely he had been throughout his childhood. He said that he was brought up to think you were not a man if you were in touch with feelings; he became impatient and irritated if others talked too much about their feelings. He described his mother as being like a shadow – 'too busy to think about feelings'.

He started masturbating to images from the age of 11 using catalogues with women's clothes and underwear, and later accessing online pornography. From the age of 13 he started using pornography that was 'quite hard core', retreating to his room and locking the door and enjoying that it was secret. Now it was inconceivable to him to masturbate without pornography. He said that he looked at images of women with perfect bodies and imagined himself with them. Later it became clear that they had surgically enhanced, inflated, pneumatic bodies with exaggerated female characteristics. His use of pornography was only one part of his use of screens – he was unable to go to sleep without watching films or TV series on his tablet.

He was deeply afraid of commitment, of feeling trapped and of people wanting more from him than he could give. In the conflict between his longing for closeness and wanting to be alone, pornography let him control the distance – he could imagine intimacy, but it was all under his control. He said that he was afraid that if he got into a long-term relationship he would be a burden. This speaks of his feeling that the depressed, hungry, angry part of him, would sap the life out of a family.

Coen (1981), in a paper long predating the internet and internet pornography, describes how one function of masturbation in men is in providing *'the illusory presence of another person which extends to identification with the comforting mother to restore the symbiotic duality'*. We can think that it was not just a sexual partner that Liam was summoning up in his imagination, but at some level, a symbiotic relationship with a comforting mother in whom he could immerse himself, but safely, without the threat of engulfment or abandonment.

For people such as Liam, the use of screens could be thought of as a kind of electronic transitional object, conjuring a sense of the presence of another and of himself in relation to another in fantasy. The screens allow the creation of an area of illusion, as Winnicott (1953) describes, in the intermediate area between subjective reality and external reality. In infancy, the fantasy created by the infant is accepted as a piece of external reality – this thumb is the breast, or this teddy bear is both me and mother, both comforter and comforted. The creation of this area of illusion is a necessary step in coming to terms with external reality.

Greenacre (1970) suggests that Winnicott's notion of the transitional object applies in the context of good enough mothering. However, in the context of a chronically disturbed relationship to the mother, the child may have a disturbed sense of his or her own body and the relation to the other, and there may be premature eroticization. She proposes that, as early as the end of the first year or beginning of the second year of life, auto-erotic activities developing in the context of severe deprivation, combined with the anger generated in frustrating or depriving conditions, means that the transitional object may acquire the characteristics of an infantile fetish, or pave the way for the later development of a fetish. This is more the quality that we see with compulsive use of internet sex, when sexually exciting images on a screen do not just conjure up a sense of the benign comforting relationship to the other (or the mother), but are infused with the aggression and auto-erotic excitement that signal frustration and a retreat from relatedness. For some people, use of on-screen pornography is not a transitional step in coming to terms with the reality of the separateness of the other as Winnicott describes, but becomes much more like the compulsive retreat to a fetish that Greenacre writes about.

Hanna Segal's (1978) distinction between symbols and symbolic equations is useful in understanding the sterile, repetitious behaviour that can occur with people with sexual compulsions. In her view, in the depressive position, there is differentiation from the object and an awareness of loss. A symbol is then used to recreate the experience of the original object in its absence. In contrast, in the very earliest use of symbols in the paranoid schizoid position, self and other are not fully differentiated. At this level of functioning, early symbols *'are not felt to by the ego to be substitutes or symbols [for the object] but to be the object itself'* (p.164). In the depressive position the thumb that is sucked substitutes for the absent breast; in the paranoid schizoid position, it is felt to be the breast itself. In her view it is this 'symbolic equation' of the symbol and the thing itself which underpins the concrete thinking in psychosis.

In many compulsive sexual behaviours it is as though some image, some experience is sought with an absolute desperation, as though this will finally be 'the object itself' as Segal describes. In Liam's case, this was possibly the generous nurturing mother. There is a kind of concreteness to the desperation. Yet Liam looks at these images and knows that they are not the idealized mother, their bodies are not real, and their sexual responses are enacted. They are being paid to do a job. Part of the work of therapy is to mourn the original losses, to know what he yearns for and missed out on, to know that he can't ever find the perfectly luxurious mothering that he can blissfully lose himself in – and so to become dis-illusioned. Functioning at this more depressive position level, there is the possibility of enjoying a temporary retreat into fantasy, maybe the conscious use of sex or pornography – knowing it is a symbol of all that was wished for and desired in infancy, but it will never be the thing itself. It seems that his illusory search for a perfectly comforting and exciting mother gave this behaviour a kind of compulsion and desperation which kept him locked in an addictive cycle, and which caused him great shame and distress.

Returning to Glasser's (Glasser, 1979) core complex, the internet is like an idealized object that you can climb into, merge with, lose yourself in, that can apparently bear the enactment of hostile sadistic impulses as well as sexuality, and that appears to by-pass self-consciousness and shame about such impulses. What people are discovering is that the internet is not as passive and tolerant as was imagined. In fact, the mirror reflects, the drama turns nasty, and as one patient said, he felt there was a monstrous creature in a cage, and he thought he was rattling its cage through his activities on the internet, but the creature turned round and bit him.

Liam and Mano both substituted the world of illusion for the painful reality of bleak internal worlds. At the outset of therapy neither was emotionally articulate or psychologically minded but in therapy each began to bear depressive realities and acknowledge the painful loneliness of their life and patterns. At this point, their search for more manic and omnipotent excitement could begin to abate.

'Marsha': sexting and sexualization as a response to deprivation and dissociation

While those presenting with compulsive use of internet pornography are predominantly male, females often present for help having got caught up in interactive activity such as sexting (Ferree, 2003). Typical was Marsha, 13, who became involved in a sexting scenario which threatened her reputation. An only child adopted from Russia at 7 by a single mother, when young she had been both seriously neglected and exposed to sexualized behaviour. She struggled in friendships, felt lonely, emotionally flat and deadened. She managed cravings for an intimacy which she also feared by engaging in inappropriate online encounters with men, which she found exciting.

Marsha had some features often also seen in males addicted to pornography. She presented in an emotionally withdrawn, lifeless way. Her potential life-force, her 'libido', seemed only to come alive via the excitement of online encounters. Otherwise she could not express or even know that she had desires.

Marsha indulged in worrying internet activity in a way that meant she would inevitably get caught, provoking her mother who then became despairing and angry with her. This pattern became a form of sadomasochistic enactment in itself, allowing her to avoid real intimacy with her mother while keeping her mother close and 'on her case', in classic core complex style (Glasser, 1992).

After being caught posting naked pictures of herself online, her technology was removed. Ostensibly, consciously, she was pleased to be protected. However, at stressful periods, such as exam times or when a friendship went wrong, her conscious will was overridden by less conscious forces. Then she would do almost anything to acquire technology, fuelling what seemed like an addiction. She would scour the house, ghostlike in the night, find old laptops and smartphones, and communicate online with strangers.

Many men communicating with girls like Marsha are using false names, grooming several children simultaneously, yet making each child feel special and unique. The underlying issues are not new, in Marsha's case the paucity of love, attention and kindness in her early life and her early, possibly preverbal, exposure to exciting sexuality, giving rise to a personality ripe for such exploitation. However, for Marsha, as for many addicted tech users, the technology allows these vulnerable young people to be identified and to be exploited with an ease impossible in the past.

Marsha had to slowly learn to bear the feelings stirred up in intimate human encounters, including in her therapy. As more genuine emotional relating became possible, her core complex anxieties could slowly be relinquished. She could be more vulnerable, especially with her mother and therapist. She began to crave attention, and believe in its possibility, but this also felt like a huge risk. She would quickly retreat when she felt spurned or be manipulative and controlling to get the attention she craved. Therapy can be a kind of practice for life, a place to learn about emotions and one's inner life, where intimacy and trust in genuine closeness can be experimented with, and evolve.

The process of becoming emotionally healthier for young people like Marsha is slow, with many false dawns, rapidly followed by regression to former ways of managing pain. Powerful feelings of loss and need can get stirred up, as in gaps between sessions. As Marsha learnt to bear such feelings, and as hopeful aspects of her personality developed, her symptoms began to abate. As Marsha began to believe in her likeability and her ability to be known emotionally, she relied less on old patterns, her desires no longer enacted in such worrying ways.

With many pornography users, we see something similar. Addictive symptoms worsen with increased vulnerability, and in crises. What they, like Marsha, lack is a good internal object to rely on, to help them bear and come through difficulty, to help them trust that things can work out well-enough in the end. Of course, there needs to be weaning from the technology too. While someone is coming off a drug like cocaine one does not leave piles of it around their home. The same applies to the temptations of technology. Psychotherapeutic treatments may need to be supported by careful management of the environment, and equally, behavioural approaches alone may be insufficient without understanding of the dynamic and emotional issues involved.

As already discussed, worrying use of technology usually involves a turning away from challenging feeling states, from human relationships and intimacy. When the powerful emotions linked to intimacy can be borne, then addictive tendencies diminish.

'Dillon': the risks of enactment in the virtual world

Dillon's relationship with pornography was unusual. By 16 he had a conviction for the possession and distribution of indecent images of children, with all the repercussions that come with being a registered sex offender. On the surface, little about his past would have indicated serious disturbance. His history was apparently relatively straightforward, without obvious abuse or trauma, apart from mild bullying by an older half-brother, and a somewhat fraught parental divorce when he was nine years old.

Nevertheless, his sexual desires were consistently disturbed. He had never found girls or boys of his own age attractive, going cold at the thought of sexual encounters with them. He was often aroused in public situations where there were children, such as swimming baths, or on buses and trains. He was good-looking, girls his age often approached him, and he had unsuccessfully tried to become involved with them, desperately wanting to be 'normal'. He had only ever felt arousal for pre-pubescent girls, but desperately wished he was not this way.

Initially Dillon managed these feelings by looking at images online, often relatively innocuous ones, such as in clothing catalogues. Then he discovered the 'dark web', where illegal sites could be accessed. Here he found pornography depicting sexual encounters with girls of the age he was aroused by, sometimes involving overt sexual acts with adult men. This discovery left him feeling less alone and filled him with relief. Such pornography use lessened his fantasizing about real live pre-pubertal girls, but perpetuated his deviant sexual interests and left him at risk of arrest.

In DSM 5 (American Psychiatric Association, 2013), 16 is the lowest age at which a diagnosis of paedophilia can be made, and in Dillon's case it might be premature to see this as an enduring sexual interest. Recidivism rates for juvenile sex offenders are relatively low leading some to conclude that 'juveniles who commit sexual offences should not be labelled as sex offenders for life' (p.5, Lobanov-Rostovsky, 2015). Nevertheless, this is a concerning symptom in a young person. A striking aspect of Dillon's presentation was his self-hatred. With patient's presenting with paedophilic thoughts, it can take time to unravel whether this is primarily driven by libido or desire (imagining something which, however, perverse, gives them pleasure) or driven by sado-masochism (that is, making themselves imagine the worst thing they can possibly imagine and so making themselves into someone 'loathsome' (see Wood, 2014). Some people who view indecent images online, appear not to be primarily paedophilic in their sexual interests, but only seek out these materials after immersion in internet pornography leads to a breakdown in their self-control and adult sexual adaptation (Wood, 2013).

Many who undertake paedophilic acts, or have sexual fantasies about children, were abused as children or inappropriately exposed to high levels of sexual stimulation. Imagining or viewing sexual enactments towards children can represent a revisiting of their own troubled history, or a projection into children of aspects of themselves they wish to disown, or a projective reversal, a wish to witness someone else being abused and helpless, as they once were. One late adolescent patient had been using ordinary pornography for some years but found himself gripped in his late teens by the temptation to click onto links that led him to pornographic images of children. During his therapy, he was able to link this to abuse he had suffered from an uncle and a cousin when still a pre-schooler. Often, if such initial traumas are worked through in therapy, and links made to when and why their feelings and impulses are triggered, the re-enactments lessen. Many people who were abused as children, in adulthood nevertheless relate sexually to people of their own age.

In Dillon's therapy, we did not arrive at a full understanding of his sexuality and why it had become so fixed on children. There was no apparent history of sexual abuse, but sometimes in longer-term therapy it becomes clear how, even without explicit sexual intrusion, the child or young person has turned to sexual excitement as a way of dealing with emotional trauma and this develops into a fixation on childhood sexuality. The age of the child who becomes of sexual interest is often the age of maximal emotional trauma for the individual growing up. It was not possible to explore such areas with Dillon because, even though he worked hard in therapy, there were limits to what could be achieved in once-weekly therapy which was terminated when he moved away. Nevertheless, exploring his sexual fantasies and the body sensations he experienced, both when anxious and when aroused, over time yielded significant results. He became much less self-punitive and came to understand that thoughts could pass through his mind without him acting on them. Discovering that he could actively ground himself by focusing on his body-states was liberating and transformational.

Dillon eventually left therapy to go to University confident that he could manage in the outside world, less plagued by self-hatred and shame.

Conclusions

The dangers posed by digital technology are much higher for vulnerable children. More fortunate children have emotionally sensitive attachment figures who can empathize with them, helping to manage difficult experiences such as frustration or anxiety, promoting self-regulation, empathy and emotional regulation (Kochanska and Kim, 2012). In the adolescent period, this capacity for self-understanding, acceptance and emotion regulation will facilitate the tasks of coming to terms with the sexual body, and the challenges of exploring sexual intimacy and the establishment of a sexual identity. Those who have rarely been empathized with tend to struggle to regulate emotions, and are more vulnerable to the lure of technology as a way of seeming to manage or avoid difficult emotions.

A psychoanalytic perspective invites exploration of what the internet offers not only to the conscious mind, but also to the unconscious. Some will be more drawn by the allure of internet sex than others, such as those who have been physically, sexually or emotionally abused, those who have been isolated or neglected, those who struggle with intimacy, as well as those who were inappropriately stimulated sexually in childhood.

For those with such vulnerabilities, the internet can contribute to a breakdown of defences and an increase in more manic, narcissistic, perverse and sadistic ways of relating to imagined 'others' on the internet, and this can come to disrupt and dominate mental functioning. Yet in psychoanalytic psychotherapy, as seen in some of these cases, as the inner world changes, virtual sex can lose its allure. Central to such change are the very real challenges of managing a real world relationship with an other in the transference; challenging for the patient who fears intimacy, and challenging for the therapist who must often bear the projection into them of the inadequacy or depression that cannot be tolerated. This inevitably is slow and painstaking work in which the therapist provides a way of relating which can ultimately offer an alternative to the immediate excitement and gratification offered by the virtual world.

References

American Psychiatric Association. (2013). *Diagnostic and statistical manual of mental disorders*. 5th ed. Arlington, VA: American Psychiatric Association.

Bollas, C. (2000) *Hysteria*. London, Routledge.

Brand, M., Snagowski, J., Laier, C. & Maderwald, S. (2016) Ventral striatum activity when watching preferred pornographic pictures is correlated with symptoms of Internet pornography addiction. *NeuroImage*. 129, 224–232.

Coen, S. J. (1981) Sexualization as a predominant mode of defense. *Journal of the American Psychoanalytic Association*. 29 (4), 893–920.

Damasio, A. R. (1999) *The feeling of what happens: body, emotion and the making of consciousness*. London, Heineman.

Ferree, M. C. (2003) Women and the web: cybersex activity and implications. *Sexual and Relationship Therapy*. 18 (3), 385–393.

Fonagy, P. & Target, M. (1998) Mentalization and the changing aims of child psychoanalysis. *Psychoanalytic Dialogues*. 8 (1), 87–114.

Freud, A. (1978) The principal task of child analysis. *Bulletin of the Anna Freud Centre*. 1 (1), 11–16.

Glasser, M. (1979) Some aspects of the role of aggression in the perversions. *Sexual Deviation*. 2, 278–305.

Glasser, M. (1992) Problems in the psychoanalysis of certain narcissistic disorders. *The International Journal of Psychoanalysis*. 73 (3), 493–503.

Greenacre, P. (1970) The transitional object and the fetish with special reference to the role of illusion. *International Journal of Psycho-Analysis*. 51, 447–456.

Hamilton-Giachritis, C. D., Hanson, E., Whittle, H. & Beech, A. (2017) *Everyone deserves to be safe and happy*. NSPCC Publisher.

Kidd, D., Ongis, M. & Castano, E. (2016) On literary fiction and its effects on theory of mind. *Scientific Study of Literature*. 6 (1), 42–58.

Kochanska, G. & Kim, S. (2012) Toward a new understanding of legacy of early attachments for future antisocial trajectories: evidence from two longitudinal studies. *Development and Psychopathology*. 1 (1), 1–24.

Kraus, S. W., Voon, V. & Potenza, M. N. (2016) Neurobiology of compulsive sexual behavior: emerging science. *Neuropsychopharmacology*. 41 (1), 385–386.

Laufer, M. (1976) The central masturbation fantasy, the final sexual organization, and adolescence. *Psychoanalytic Study of the Child*. 31, 297–316.

Lobanov-Rostovsky, C. (2015) *Recidivism of juveniles who commit sexual offences*. Sex offender management assessment and planning initiative, US Dept of Justice, July 2015.

Lemma, A. (2014) An order of pure decision: growing up in a virtual world and the adolescent's experience of the body. In: Lemma, A. & Caparrotta, L. (eds.) *Psychoanalysis in the technoculture era*. Hove, East Sussex, Routledge.

Music, G. (2016) *Nurturing natures: attachment and children's emotional, social and brain development*. London, Psychology Press.

Nathanson, A. (2016) Embracing darkness: clinical work with adolescents and young adults addicted to sexual enactments. *Journal of Child Psychotherapy*. 43 (3), 272–284.

Negash, S., Sheppard, N. V. N., Lambert, N. M. & Fincham, F. D. (2016) Trading later rewards for current pleasure: pornography consumption and delay discounting. *The Journal of Sex Research*. 53 (6), 689–700.

Park, B. Y., Wilson, G., Berger, J., Christman, M., Reina, B., Bishop, F., Klam, W. P. & Doan, A. P. (2016) Is internet pornography causing sexual dysfunctions? A review with clinical reports. *Behavioral Sciences*. 6 (3), online. doi:10.3390/bs6030017.

Segal, H. (1978) On symbolism. *International Journal of Psycho-Analysis*. 59, 315–319.

Winnicott, D. W. (1953) Psychoses and child care. *British Journal of Medical Psychology*. 26 (1), 68–74.

Wood, H. (2011) The internet and its role in the escalation of sexually compulsive behaviour. *Psychoanalytic Psychotherapy*. 25 (2), 127–142.

Wood, H. (2013) Internet pornography and paedophilia. *Psychoanalytic Psychotherapy*. 27 (4), 319–338.

Wood, H. (2014) Internet offenders from a sense of guilt. In: Lemma, A. & Caparotta, L. (eds.) *Psychoanalysis in the technoculture era*. Hove, East Sussex, Routledge.

Chapter 5

Seeing and being seen: the psychodynamics of pornography through the lens of Winnicott's thought

John Woods

The excessive use of internet pornography, so easily available now, with increasingly extreme images, can cause young people to become isolated from others, alienated from reality, and psychologically harmed. In the worst cases, seen clinically, a compulsive form of voyeurism means that the young person is so full of shame he cannot bear to be seen and becomes painfully alone with his violent masturbation fantasies. Something has happened to their psychosexual development which may be elucidated by the ideas of D.W. Winnicott. For instance he described how the ability to be in a sexual relationship that is 'ego-related', i.e. one in which two people have the possibility of love depends, upon a maturational process that paradoxically leads to 'the capacity to be alone'. This process in his view flows from, feelings aroused by the primal scene: 'the excited relationship between the parents....is accepted by the child who is healthy and able to master the hate...' (Winnicott, 1958b:p.31). He went on to discuss the consequent development of a good internal object as dependent on the acquisition of genital potency, the corresponding female role and the ability of the child to identify with each of the parents. What we find in cases of psychological damage exacerbated by excessive pornography is the destruction of this process of personality development.

At the Portman Clinic, London, psychological treatment is offered to young people and adults whose offences and other problems are frequently linked to the sexual imagery available over the internet. They sometimes report being impelled to commit sexual assaults by the compulsive use of this imagery to feed masturbation fantasies. Though it goes against the grain to impute responsibility for sexual crimes to the media, there are recent reports of judgements which take the influence of pornography as a mitigating factor in cases of sexual offences by young people. For example Judge Gareth Hawkesworth in 2012 gave a community order to a 14-year-old boy found guilty of raping a five-year-old girl, saying, 'I'm satisfied that the rape was impulsive and I believe you have become sexualized by exposure to the corruption of pornography. It was the fault of society' (Avery, 2012). If so, we may ask, what is society doing about this?

Even more questionable messages are being given to young people about illegal images of child sexual abuse, which are trailed before every pornography user, access to which is completely unrestricted. This is one of the reasons why internet pornography is qualitatively different from previous forms of pornography (Wood, 2007). When the police are able to track such content over the internet many young people are astonished to find themselves in deep trouble for 'just looking' as they see it. They come to us with criminal convictions, and not surprisingly are confused by contradictory messages from adult society, which condones the supply of such perverse stimulation into the world of childhood. It is as if we are punishing the child who buys drugs at the school gate, ignoring the supplier. It would be hard to find a more blatant example of the 'antisocial act' of the adolescent that reflects the failure of the (adult) environment (Winnicott, 1958a). Society seems to be saying, 'Look all you like at all these highly stimulating things, normally forbidden; get sexually aroused, but if you look at *this* particular stuff the law will come down hard on you'.

The harm being done by internet pornography

Referrals to the Portman for the problematic use of pornography have increased dramatically in recent years, so that many patients come with such problems. Similarly, relationship counsellors report that the use of internet pornography is a cause of tension and conflict for as many as half of their clients seeking help with marital and/or sexual problems (Paul, 2006). Whereas many people have a 'take it or leave it' response to pornography, (as with other potentially dangerous substances, alcohol, tobacco etc.), others fall foul of a compulsive reaction and their lives are seriously affected (Wood, 2013:p.101).

Because of growing numbers of these referrals the Portman took the unprecedented step of joining with the British Broadcasting Corporation in a survey of young men (18–24) and their use of pornography. A quarter of them were worried about the amount of pornography they watch on the internet. Heavy users were more likely to report problems with their jobs, relationships and sex lives. They were not having more fun but were worried about themselves and what they were looking at, and reported more relationship problems (Wood, 2013).

A landmark in this field is the Manning Report (2005) to the US Senate, 'Pornography's Impact on Marriage & The Family', which brought together evidence from many sources. Studies reported increased marital distress, risk of separation and divorce, and increasing numbers of people struggling with compulsive and addictive sexual behaviour; also many negative effects on children, including traumatic emotional responses, earlier onset of first sexual intercourse, increased incidence of sexually transmitted diseases, increased risk for developing sexually addictive behaviour (Manning, 2005; Owens et al., 2012).

In the UK, a special parliamentary committee, chaired by Claire Perry, found that the scale of exposure is so vast that four out of five 16-year-olds regularly access pornography online, the average age of first internet exposure to pornography is 11 years of age, and the largest group of users are 12 to 17 years of age (www.claireperry.org.uk). It means that any child who is curious about sex can tap that word into a search engine, and instantly have access to thousands of graphic videos.

Research has demonstrated the effects of this process: studies of ordinary adolescents (college students) have found that the relationship between exposure to sexually explicit media is linked with notions of women as sex objects (Peter & Valkenburg, 2007). Risk-taking behaviours, such as unprotected sex, and increased anal and oral intercourse, were more frequent in a sample of young men who had high use of internet pornography (Häggström-Nordin et al., 2005). Susan Greenfield (2002) notes a relaxation of boundaries against sexual violence and that ordinary young men feel that pornography has an impact on their sexual behaviour; 'they got inspired'. Girls are beginning to report how their relationships are being affected, often required to perform the kind of extreme acts that male partners are watching (Carey, 2011). Studies of Juvenile sex offenders show that the more aggressive and violent assaults are committed by boys who regularly watch internet pornography (Alexy, 2009).

Children in therapy report that these images can be deeply traumatizing; the pornography concentrates on adult sexual organs, often in acts of penetration, and presents a mechanical kind of sexual activity, devoid of human or personal interaction. They are likely to keep this secret from parents, much as children do when they are being actually sexually abused, because of fear and shame. Initially, shocked and horrified, the child is confused that the adult world has made this private world so easily available to them. The child goes into adolescence assuming, for example, that women always want sex and that sex is nothing to do with relationships. There is no indication in internet pornography of how a couple might negotiate a relationship, let alone resolve conflict or establish intimacy. The viewer is shown that men can have whomever they want and that women respond the way men want them to. Anal and oral sex are the norms; perpetual female orgasm is to be expected. The man's erection is never ending, until he ejaculates, usually over the woman's face, often with a group of other men doing the same. Offensive as this might be to read or hear, I think we have to recognize what our children are being subjected to.

For many young boys, this means their first sexual experience does not begin with a nervous request to meet or get to know someone, it is watching a parade of degrading images of women, who only want sex, often mixed in with violent abuse. It is important to recognize that these images are being watched in a state of sexual arousal and masturbation, thus ensuring a powerful association between the two.

'James', 15, referred after a caution for indecent assault on a five-year-old boy, admitted to a fascination with internet pornography, and 'wanted to know what sex felt like'. The younger child was the only available sexual object, he thought. He did not imagine that someone being penetrated sexually should give consent, since, as he said 'they always want it on the Internet'. Though he was made aware he had 'crossed a line' as the child protection team put it, he had little sense of having done harm. It took him a year in therapy to make a connection between the offence and his anger with his parents, preoccupied as they were with their professional lives.

In the case of 'Jeremy', (14) police arrived at his home because they identified that someone was accessing illegal images of child sexual abuse. It emerged that for more than three years, Jeremy had been visiting pornographic websites for hours every night, while his parents assumed he was using his computer for homework. Even when his school performance began to suffer, they had no idea of the perverse world the shy, quiet boy was inhabiting while upstairs in his bedroom. He recounted the development of his compulsion: 'I stopped leaving my room and seeing friends because when I was away from the pornography, I was dying to get back to see what else I could find'.

Deeply ashamed, he said convincingly that he had not set out to find extreme images which then became fascinating. 'Websites led to others and I was looking at weird stuff I could never have imagined – animals, children, stabbing, strangling'. He described how away from the screen he would be tormented by the images. He would return to the computer to get them 'out there' on to the screen, but in watching again, they were reinforced in his mind. He was glad that he was made to stop, but still feared he may never form a healthy relationship – 'It`s like pervert is written across my forehead. It makes me think I might never have a proper girlfriend – the pictures still come back making me want to shout, "Stop, stop." But they won't go away'.

It is becoming increasingly common that girls are induced to display their body sexually over the internet; for example 'Jemma', age 14, was referred by social workers because she was displaying her body and masturbating for the web camera, enticing men not only to watch but to arrange meetings. The men were breaking the law, but the authorities had no idea what to do about Jemma. In an assessment she said she was doing this 'for fun', that it was only what she had seen grown women do, and she got a 'buzz' out of the attention she was getting. There were promises of rewards from men but she said she had no real intention of meeting them. We asked if she could see the harm she was doing, even to herself? She complained of her life being 'boring', which could also be understood as her experiencing a fear of depression. She had no friends; they were 'stupid'. She had already ignored several warnings from teachers and social workers about her use of the internet, but it seemed she could not bear to give up the excitement she could create in others and herself. She could not see that the pleasure of using her sexuality to get men into serious trouble might have anything to do with the protracted, bitter and at times violent separation her parents were going through. Some therapeutic work might have led to some progress in these areas but she firmly declined it.

Psychodynamic aspects of compulsive behaviour

The escalating behaviour that results from compulsive use of pornography seems to derive from some digging down, as it were, into deeper layers of the personality, uncovering impulses and desires that hitherto have been dormant or would otherwise remain so (Wood, 2007, 2013). Wood points out how the stimulus of certain imagery taps into previously unconscious content, penetrating layers of more developmentally appropriate defences in the personality. The internet stimulates manic defences of its own, especially in those more vulnerable to emotional stress and deprivation; anything seems possible, there is the illusion of invisibility, and apparent permission given to previously forbidden desires (Wood, 2013). Whilst it seems unlikely that the internet creates specific sexual interests afresh, Wood finds through clinical work that it may have acted as a catalyst, releasing traits which would otherwise remain hidden, unconscious and possibly unrealized. These may reflect emotionally charged childhood fantasies about bodies, intercourse, violence and associated anxieties. Childhood curiosity is both stimulated and instantly gratified. Infantile sexual fantasies are released, and generate their own reality. Connections are made with unconscious contents via this imagery, which may include for some people the after-effects of their own abuse, or primitive theories about bodies and body function. Anal or oral theories about where babies come from are mixed in with primitive fears of sexual intercourse as violent or annihilatory. A regression is set in motion, that may be translated into action. Ordinary defences are bypassed, just as the belief in external reality is washed away. Traumatic elements are exposed but the excitement results in a compulsion to repeat the traumatic scenario in an active sexual form, in order to overcome the helplessness of trauma. The world of illusion and the screen has failed as infantile anxieties return, pushing for re-enactment, sometimes in the form of sexual aggression against the body of another.

Unrestricted access to internet pornography undermines normal development. Ordinarily, a child learns to cope with limits, especially of access to the object of desire. Instead he or she is now being offered fantasies in which omnipotently they can have anything and everything they want, without restraint or prohibition. Thus, a child and even more, an adolescent loses the capacity to deal with frustration or delay gratification. The flow of sexual imagery taps into what Winnicott, drawing on Freud (1918) was referring to above as the Primal Scene, that is, the child's conception of parental intercourse, a template for sexual relations. In the usual course of events, the child has to deal with being excluded from the parental intercourse and copes with that loss. He or she accepts the difference between the sexes, and between the generations. The child moves away from incestuous bonds, eventually to form his or her own relationships. But with the artificially induced voyeurism of endless pornography the child comes to believe he need never give up the original object of desire in fantasy – not only does he see what adults do, he participates by his own sexual activity, masturbation, and can identify with either sex, in any position, in all senses; he is in danger of failing to develop a separate adult sexual identity. Voyeurism can take such a hold it becomes a substitute for real sexual relationship, though ultimately leading of course to disappointment. Here is a very different experience from the looking at and 'creating' each other in Winnicott's theory of 'object presenting', Winnicott (1971). As Khan also observes 'one technique the pervert uses against disillusionment is to strive after *intensity* of erotic experiences. This intensity is the pervert's equivalent for object relating' (Khan, 1969:p.563).

The case of 'Martin'

Aged 17, Martin was becoming socially phobic; with a history of refusing school because of being bullied he was referred by a social worker who had been trying to get him out of the house. Father had never been in the picture. Mother remained single, working to support herself and her son, and feeling helpless in the face of his withdrawal from the world. The referrer worried that excessive use of the internet was exacerbating Martin's social phobia. Persuaded to attend, for 'at least one session', by the social worker, he admitted to worries about his increasingly compulsive and time consuming use of internet pornography, with increasingly violent imagery. These he felt were invading his life even at times when not hooked into the screen. Initially relieved at having someone to talk to, he found himself agreeing to give therapy 'a try for a few weeks'. Soon, however, he was experiencing painful feelings about his life, and especially that the therapist was as indifferent and contemptuous as he believed his father to be. Treatment at this point depended on the support of the social worker who had in the meantime also managed to get Martin onto a work/study experience.

Grudgingly, a few weeks later he reported progress regarding work and studies, and that life was 'a bit less meaningless' than he had averred. And suddenly a new development occurred; he encountered a girl at his work placement whom he really liked. There was tremendous anxiety at his sexual desires for her. 'She could never like me', he insisted. In any case, he said, there were rules forbidding him to talk to her. She was due to leave the scheme soon, and he fretted about how he might approach her. Almost as an aside he mentioned he was not looking at pornography much. The girl at work became the preoccupation. His therapist interpreted this idealization, that as bad as he felt himself to be, so he was putting all the good into her. There was still anger towards the therapy, but less desperation. It was interesting that he had created a situation where there was a real boundary, unlike the internet where there appears to be no limits. Gloomily he regarded it as always his fate that he would never get anywhere with girls. He would always be the one 'left with the crap', but the way he communicated this had changed. He seemed to be at a point where he felt the need for a good father figure. He felt sure that any girl would be disgusted with him if she knew his 'dirty thoughts'. The therapist commented that he imagined this to be her judgement, but actually it was his self disgust, and need to change.

Martin was perhaps on the brink of a capacity to be alone: '...the impulse having arrived, the id experience can be fruitful, and the object can be a part or the whole of the attendant person, namely the mother ... (and) the infant can have an experience which feels real. A large number of such experiences form the basis for a life that has reality in it instead of futility' (Winnicott, 1958b:p.34).

When the girl did not respond to his messages, he was less devastated than expected (by either of us), and said 'it's tough, but I can get over it'. He went on to say that he no longer found the pornography interesting. 'Something has changed. It's.... boring. I think if I were to go back to that I would have lost'. It seemed there was now a shift in his psychic functioning; he had found a limit, an oedipal situation, not an universe where everything was apparently permitted.

Of course further setbacks, alternating, hopefully, with further advances should be anticipated. But the material thus far has shown salient points of adolescent crisis, sexual conflict, and perverse fantasies. His development before treatment had stalled, and his regressive breakdown in the face of adolescent emotional stress was made more dangerous by internet pornography. Regression to mental states of omnipotence, splitting and projection is made easy by the internet. How many young people are there who, lacking that conscientious social worker, and the knowledge that help exists, are lost in cyberspace?

In a later session Martin was complaining about being tired from his work, and at home by his mother's needs. 'I escape to my room, my zone. God, what would I do without my zone?'

'To look at pornography?' His therapist asked.

He looked blank. 'What? Oh that, I've given up all that. I can't be bothered with that. No I just need rest, I'm exhausted'. He looked tolerantly as though this therapist needed to catch up.

Discussion

The internet is of course not only destructive in its effects but also the lack of regulation magnifies the dangers that exist certainly for some, (who knows

how many), consumers. And pornography is not the only pitfall; the gla-
mour and excitement of celebrity culture, made omnipresent by the internet,
are both tantalizing and isolating for many adolescents, and there is no
protection for those even more exposed to the websites that are encouraging
self harm, depression, or gender dysphoria, without any regard for individual needs. With internet pornography the intensity of the masturbatory
sexual experience begins to substitute for ordinary (or real) sexual relationships. The more someone engages in the process of looking, whilst in a
state of high arousal, the fear of being looked at, or being seen, becomes
greater. There is a break between the subject and the viewed object. The
object viewed over the internet usually cannot see the subject. In the case of
Jemma, (above), there was a different break; she could let herself be seen, in
certain carefully controlled ways, producing an impact, but not seeing, or
owning, those effects. The task of therapy would be to re-establish these
links.

Mother and baby usually look into each other's eyes; the baby sees itself,
in the mother's lively reflection of the baby, (Winnicott, 1967). In this exchange between self and other, there is a development of emotional resonance, positive reflection and security. Delay or inhibition of this process
produces a lack of emotional resonance, absence of autonomy and excessive
fear of the outer world. Wright (1991) explores the development of self in the
eyes of the object when he writes that, 'The space of self consciousness arises
around the subject, as the child becomes aware of the looking of the object.
It is the space within which the person looks at himself through the eyes of
the other' (1991:p.xiii). What happens to the person who cannot bear to be
seen, but only to look?

In the world of internet pornography, the aggression inherent in the
looking provokes a terror of being seen, and shamed. The looker is given
power, apparently, to see anything and everything, with or without consent.
But the terror of being seen, and shamed is increased because of the projection of hostility. Wright (1991) goes on to define shame as the experience
of being looked at by the other who can see things not available to the self,
giving rise to the question whether the self that it now is for the other will
still be loved. This is a crisis for the shamed person, and can become a
fulcrum in psychotherapy. In normal development, there is a working
through of shame and fear of exposure of forbidden thoughts, towards
maturation and differentiation from the primary object. For someone stuck
in their development this incomplete process can be recovered in
psychotherapy.

The first few months of therapy saw Martin attempting to recreate a
protected space where he could avoid being challenged, as he had by his
avoidance of social situations. Shame at revealing hidden aspects of himself,
those he felt were 'outside the norm', as he put it, produced anger, sometimes a contemptuous attitude towards the therapist, momentary feelings of

despair, and quick attempts to cover up but Martin's voyeurism was primarily a symptom of self disgust. Inevitably, the therapy brought him into contact with parts of the self previously denied. He had been hiding behind a grandiose view of himself, but began to see that this defence was at the cost of isolation both from the external world and his own needs. At adolescence the compulsion had not crystallized into a true addiction, and so he could make use of the opportunity to make contact with someone, perhaps at first the social worker, and then a therapist, whose closeness became bearable. He began to drop the distorted sense of himself and uncover his 'dirty thoughts'. This process took place in relation to the idea of woman, which he could see he had objectified, dehumanized, and therefore made unavailable to him. A different idea, of a relationship with an actual woman could be formed within the context of the transference in which the therapist was not only the helpful father he would hardly have believed possible but also as the hated and hating father who could now be tolerated. He encountered a real boundary at work with an object of his desire, and by accepting it he also created a boundary between his fantasy and reality.

Winnicott (1967) defined psychotherapy as 'seeing': 'Even when our patients do not get healed they are grateful to us for seeing them as they are, and this gives satisfaction of a deep kind' (Winnicott, 1967:pp.117–118). Being seen became for Martin an antidote to his voyeurism. No longer was he in a perverse dyad with his screen/debased sexual mother. The therapist became a third element in his world, which could represent or mediate external reality, though the path to the door of the clinic had to be cleared, and maintained by the referring social worker. Through this means external reality became preferable to the pseudo reality of electronic media. As it happened in this case there was no direct contact with the social worker, but he was very much around in our discussion, as a representative of the external world, and used by Martin to help negotiate his fear of failure and humiliation.

To turn now to the world outside the psychotherapists consulting room – it has to be asked why are we turning a blind eye to the very damaging effects of internet pornography in our society?

The therapist in the social world

After the recent scandal in the UK at the sexual abuse by the entertainer, Jimmy Savile, for so long ignored by the authorities, we have to ask how it is that the sexual abuse of children can go on in plain sight, and for decades not be 'noticed'. Is there something we do not wish to recognize in ourselves? It is not enough to say as in Savile Report that he 'groomed a nation' (National Society for the Prevention of Cruelty to Children & Metropolitan Police, 2013) because we are not vulnerable children to fall under the sway of a calculating abuser. It is interesting that so many said after the revelations, 'but I always thought he was a creep'. How do we account for the many disclosures that came to nothing because they were ignored or discounted? If this occurred in a family, or some smaller institution than the BBC or NHS, then we would assume collusion, and would ask, what is the investment in this abuse for the apparently innocent bystander? Is there a vicarious gratification at large in seeing the corruption of youth? Like the predatory paedophile, do we envy the beauty and innocence of childhood so that we allow and even unconsciously take pleasure in its spoliation? The abuser may be treated with contempt, but perhaps this conceals envy of his freedom to act. When he is exposed and pilloried the moral outrage perhaps covers a secret satisfaction at the punishment of someone who is now identified as the one who has stolen the forbidden fruit of infantile sexuality.

'It's not our business', the psychotherapist may say, 'our job is to treat patients'. The trouble with that, to my mind, is that we are merely patching up the few cases we are in a position to treat, and ignoring the root of the problem. It is as if we were treating a handful of individuals with a disease like cholera or typhoid, not noticing the infected source of water. Internet pornography is in that sense a Public Health issue. Whilst we do not have a vaccine, there are preventative measures that as psychotherapists we can engage with. The Manning Report concluded that government should take a lead in implementing technological solutions that separate internet content, allowing consumers to choose the type of legal content, in educating the public about the risks of pornography consumption, and supporting research that examines aspects of internet pornography (Manning, 2005). Little of this has been done, either in the USA or in the UK. And when government fails in its duty, we have to speak truth to power.

Psychotherapists could be more active in supporting the interventions recommended by Manning in order to provide a better holding environment for children. The ideal of free expression and no censorship has to be questioned. We should alert government and commercial agencies that are responsible for regulation to the destructive power of internet pornography on children. We can contribute to organizations like the UK Council for Child Internet Safety, the Internet Watch Foundation and Safer Media that campaign, support research and are eager to learn from the specialized knowledge that mental health professionals have. The psychodynamic case has been has been substantiated by powerful legal and moral arguments (Nair, 2015) but still the government is paralysed. Is it just the libertarian discomfort with the 'nanny state' that would undermine the rights and responsibilities of parents (for this is objection always made at discussion level, especially at conferences on the subject) or is it the powerful financial interests of internet service providers that cause a blind eye to be turned? The objections based on a desire for free speech and fear of censorship need to be countered by the evidence of the harm that results from lack of regulation.

At a more ordinary level, we can support parents to monitor what images their children are exposed to and help them be firm when they feel uncomfortable about what their children are seeing. We can engage with organizations such as school and youth groups to address these issues actively, and ensure that children have a clear message about what is acceptable as against what they themselves ultimately know is wrong.

Psychotherapists need to connect with society, and take the risk of disapproval, if they are to remain relevant to human lives. In a paper about the development of maturity Winnicott remarks that 'we get left with certain social conditions and this is a legacy that we have to accept, and if necessary, alter. It is this that we eventually hand down to those who come after us' (Winnicott, 1963:pp.83–84).

References

Alexy, E. M. (2009) Pornography use as a marker for an aggressive pattern of behavior among sexually reactive children & adolescents. *Journal of the American Psychiatric Nurses Association.* 14, 442–453.

Avery, C. (2012) Boy who raped girl of 5 spared jail as judge says 'it's society's fault'. Tuesday 3 July, Metro. Quoted on www.mumsnet.com

Carey, T. (2011) *Where has my little girl gone?* London, Lion Books.

Freud, S. (1918) From the history of an infantile neurosis. *S. E.* 18. London, Hogarth.

Greenfield, S. (2002) *The private life of the brain.* London, Penguin.

Häggström-Nordin, E., Hanson, U. & Tydén, T. (2005) Associations between pornography, consumption and sexual practices among adolescents in Sweden. *International Journal of STD & AIDS.* 16, 102–107.

Khan, M. R. (1969) Role of the 'Collated Internal Object' in perversion-formations. *The International Journal of Psychoanalysis.* 50, 555–565.

Manning J. (2005) Pornography's impact on marriage & the family. Report to the US Senate. Available from: http://www.heritage.org/Research/Family/upload/852 73_1.pdf

Nair, A. (2015) *The regulation of internet pornography.* London, Routledge.

National Society for the Prevention of Cruelty to Children & Metropolitan Police (2013) *Giving victims a voice report. Metropolitan Police Service.* Retrieved 11 January 2013.

Owens, E. W., Behun, R. J., Manning, J. & Reid, R. J. (2012) The impact of internet pornography on adolescents: a review of the research. *Sexual Addiction & Compulsivity: The Journal of Treatment & Prevention.* 19, 99–122.

Peter, J. & Valkenburg, P. (2007) Adolescents' exposure to a sexualised media environment and their notions of women as sex objects. *Sex Roles.* 56, 381–395.

Paul, P. (2006) *Pornified: how porn is damaging our lives, our relationships, and our families.* US, St Martin 's Griffin.

Perry, C. (2012) *Online safety.* Available from: www.claireperry.org.uk

Winnicott, D. W. (1958a) The antisocial tendency. In: *Through paediatrics to psychoanalysis.* London, Hogarth 1975. pp. 306–315.

Winnicott, D. W. (1958b) The capacity to be alone. In: *The maturational processes and the facilitating environment*. London, Hogarth 1976. pp. 20–36.

Winnicott, D. W. (1963) From dependence towards independence in the development of the individual. In: *The maturational processes and the facilitating environment*. London, Hogarth 1976.

Winnicott, D.W. (1967) Mirror-role of mother and family in child development'. In: *The predicament of the family: a psycho-analytical symposium*. London, Hogarth.

Winnicott, D. W. (1971) The use of an object and relating through identifications. In: *Playing and reality*. London, Tavistock 1971. pp. 86–94.

Wood, H. (2007) The compulsive use of virtual sex and internet pornography. In: Morgan, D. & Rusczynski, S. (eds.) Lectures *on violence, perversion & delinquency; the portman papers*. London, Karnac.

Wood, H. (2013) The nature of sex addiction and paraphilias. In: Bower, M., Hale, R. & Wood, H. (eds.) *Addictive states of mind*. London, Karnac.

Wright, K. (1991) *Vision and separation*. London, Free Association Books.

Chapter 6

Working with mental hackers and backroom thinkers

Ariel Nathanson

Andy, now 27, described himself as having a criminal mind from a young age. Aged 15, he was at the height of his manipulative grooming success. He knew exactly which boy to approach for sex in his boarding school, and how to do it. Being very popular, he would first select a boy who seemed to hover around the inner social circle but never be allowed in. He would befriend him, and as he described, 'go to him…keep him out but make him feel that I was about to let him in with the popular boys'. In the next stage he started talking to the boy about sex with girls, maybe even look at pornography together. He described how this was an important stage in the grooming process because it created sexual excitement while being together. The third stage was more physical; it started with 'taking turns masturbating in the bathroom to the same images', and later putting his hand on the other boy's knee, waiting, and if not rejected, sometimes over a period of days, moving on to sexual touching and masturbation.

Andy was never sexually attracted to boys or men. For him, a successful sexual act was an excited celebration of his masterful criminal mind that enabled him to gain access into someone else's body. 'I would never go with someone who asked for it', he said, 'because those boys were gay or already abused and there was no challenge. I needed to get someone to do something that they wouldn't naturally want to…'.

In many ways, Andy was no different to many other Portman patients. He was highly narcissistic, a deceptive enactor, a perpetrator, cold, callous and prone to excitement and addiction. At 27, he described himself as a sex addict, which was the overt reason he wanted treatment.

Now a young adult with a good job, Andy was highly promiscuous, an expert user of dating apps who felt he could seduce almost anyone to have sex with him. He presented himself as the potential perfect boyfriend, exciting, charismatic and with good prospects. He never dated a girl more than twice and usually had a few he was involved with in parallel. He was also addicted to pornography.

Andy had a childhood story which I have heard in variations from many Portman patients. He said that his father was very successful financially but 'a pathetic man who was hardly ever there'. He and his mother were highly contemptuous of the father and would go on extravagant shopping trips to 'spend his money'. Mother was emotionally unstable and relied on Andy for closeness and comfort. They were 'best friends' until Andy discovered sex in his very early adolescence. At that point, quite abruptly, mother had a breakdown and Andy was placed in a boarding school.

When thinking about Andy's presentation from a theoretical point of view, he clearly displayed a familiar picture. He was unable to successfully mitigate the core complex (Glasser, 1979), leaving him with high level of core complex anxieties that had to be managed through enactment. He needed to control an over-intrusive, engulfing maternal object whilst keeping his own aggressive impulses at bay. The solution was probably the active participation in an exciting, oversexualized relationship with mother, which he might have felt in control of. This later developed to sexualizing other relationships in an omnipotent and exploitative way.

Andy's presentation also fitted some of Meltzer's (1992) ideas about the claustrum and life in projective identification. Andy could be described as living in projective identification with some kind of marketing director, constantly motivated to clamber to the top and trample over others as he did so. He could market his way into anything and more specifically into any-body (i.e. any-body), male or female.

Andy was callous, unemotional and virtually guilt free. He presented in therapy as wishing to gain more control over a behaviour that he felt was 'getting a bit out of hand'. If he was able to 'tone it down', as he said, he would be 'happy to get on', although, as he quickly added, 'I know that you might say that I'm an addict and I need to give it all up'. Giving it all up was said with a smile, an obvious never.

As Anne Alvarez points out in this book and elsewhere (2012), this type of presentation covers up a very barren and empty landscape, extremely depressing, that is defended against by a highly contemptuous presentation in which parents, adults and in this case, almost everybody else, is to be fooled and triumphed over.

As I started treating Andy I felt on familiar grounds. I had the theory firmly in mind, adding to the clear expectation and experience of working with patients who enact their difficulties, often as perpetrators. As a Portman clinician (Campbell, 1994), I looked for the details of the enactment – the narrative presented at the start of this chapter – noticed the excitement and the triumph, and then tried to make sense of the relational meaning, making comments and interpretations.

There was a familiar pull to enact in the sessions by smiling back when Andy described his triumphs and to join him in his misogynistic celebrations when he talked about his app-related serial conquests. However, there was also something I have not paid much attention to previously – a strong sense that Andy was looking at me from behind his eyes, carefully prescribing information and measuring my responses to his stories and descriptions. It felt as if I was being hacked into with the task of finding out something without being noticed. I thought that Andy was trying to figure out whether I was working according to some kind of a plan, leading him somewhere, obviously for his own good but without him knowing. His method was to talk about specific issues whilst carefully monitoring my reaction. For example, he spoke about feelings and emotions in order to see if I was trying to make him feel more. At other times, he spoke about what he did, gradually divulging more information that painted him as callous and cruel, seeing if he could shock me or induce a judgemental or punitive response.

Andy had a mental backroom (a concept that I shall elaborate within this chapter) from which he was constantly hacking into my mind, unable to be a patient in the same way that he was never able to be a son, a pupil, a student, a boyfriend, or a member of a group.

I spoke to Andy in a straightforward way about having a mental backroom and being a mind-hacker, which he responded to with some excitement as if enjoying being noticed for his talents after so many years of operating in the shadows. The backroom became a central concept in Andy's therapy. It put him in touch with both his omnipotence, which he thrived on, and the gaps in his relational life – never being able to be emotionally present in the here-and-now of any relationship. I was then able to talk to him about the 'risks' of intimacy and the ingenious solution he has developed in order to overcome that problem. Slowly but surely, the backroom transformed from a fantastic and colourful control centre to quite a dark place that Andy was addicted to operating from, unable to give up his position and the highs of excitement that came with it. This was very depressing to notice and induced a crisis in which the backroom started failing for the first time. It also gave Andy a chance to develop a more honest way of being in the world.

The backroom became central to the way I started thinking about many other patients presenting in different ways. Some similar to Andy, and others quite different in their relational histories, their enactments and the backroom cultures they presented. What they all had in common was the backroom structure – the capacity to hack into reality and relationships, observer, prescribe, hide and control. This chapter is about these patients, the backroom and the clinical implications of working with patients who have one.

The patients I describe here are all males, either adolescents or young adults. Although I have come across female backroom operators, I have chosen not to describe them here or discuss the differences between the sexes in order to maintain a focus on the internal structure. In many ways, this chapter is about describing initial findings that require further elaboration.

General formulation

The backroom is not unconscious. It is a hiding place in the conscious mind, part of a narcissistic structure that celebrates its own omnipotent power and accumulates it. As in Andy's case and many others, some backroom highs are experienced at the end of a grooming process when hacking is achieved and internal control of the object is experienced. Using the hack is indeed exciting and addictive but mainly because it provides a kind of a trophy or evidence to the sophistication of the process preceding it.

The backroom functions as both a hiding place and a control centre. The front room, the place people relate from in the here-and-now of every relationship, is often quite atrophied or operates mostly as a decoy, a carefully constructed front-reception to hide behind and prescribe from.

The backroom should be differentiated from the natural idea of privacy; not everything is or should be visible or communicated to others. All people have 'social selves' – the flexibility to fit into different social situations whilst holding on to a core sense of who they are. This includes the capacity to lie and even manipulate but unlike a backroom structure, it is very situational. People would act to fit into a group, for example, but remain aware of the tension between wanting to fit-in, to being different or even not belonging. They are able to tolerate this, move between belonging and not belonging and keep a healthy tension between the two.

In contrast, those with a backroom organization feel in control of the group around them like a hidden puppeteer blending into the shadows of the backstage. They might pretend to take part and be one of many but actually assume a secretive highly omnipotent position, often contemptuous, with a large part of their selves consciously concealed. They peek from behind their eyes, curtain-twitching, pretend to share a point of view but actually survey their real and relational surroundings, collect information, analyse and then prescribe to others, feeling that in doing so they control the outcome.

A young teaching assistant in a PRU, for example, described one of the students as not fitting in because he was compliant, sensitive and well behaved. However, as she later discovered, he has been secretly collating information about her for many weeks; he knew where she lived, what her apartment looked like, what her dog's name was, who was her boyfriend, and the fact that her brother died from cancer a few years earlier. Most of the information was collected from bits of conversations with her colleagues, online investigation and a picture she once naively showed him when she felt that they shared an intimate moment together. At the time, the boy made up a story and told her that his grandfather died, describing his house and the items he loved there. In response the TA shared that her brother died too and showed the boy a picture of him sitting in her flat, just before he got ill. When the boy looked at the picture he did not focus on the brother. Instead, typically for a backroom operator, he quickly surveyed the background –

the interior of the flat, secretly filing in the information. When enough information was amassed, he shocked her with his knowledge about her life, made her feel 'hacked into', taunting and cruel in using what he knew.

This boy is another example of the power of the backroom as a solution to issues with intimacy and closeness; his conscious hack allowed for an unconscious projection of his needs, which were then honestly experienced by the TA as intimacy, inducing her concern and closeness. The hacker, now aware of and excited by being in control of his victim, was able denigrate and dismiss the need for care and attachment, mocking those who experience it as gullible weak fools.

Types of backroom presentations

Although different, all backroom patients share the common denominator of secretly operating from the back of their minds. However, the origins of the backroom constellation, its internal culture and the personality organization it is part of might be quite different.

For example, not all backroom patients are callous and cruel although their actual real deprivation has almost always been hidden, camouflaged and marketed as something completely different. The level of deprivation can differ too; some backroom patients were their parents' special child, often an only child, the one with the biggest room in the house, the loft or just next to the parents, in phantasy always there, part of everything or secretly observing. Others might have been overtly and severely traumatized, living in care, some even developing a backroom already in the context of managing institutional environments.

Below I describe some distinct backroom cultures. However, they should be seen as variations on the same theme, all aspects of any backroom culture but taking different forms of focus and expression.

The voyeuristic backroom

Although voyeurism is present in every backroom constellation, some backrooms are mostly voyeuristic; Patients come across as peeking from behind their eyes and fantasizing without much active real manipulation of others. These patients might show a sort of 'reverse hacking' in which they hijack an object into their own internal fantasy, whilst maintaining a benign external presence. At other times, they might attempt to subtly impose, groom and manipulate without much real contact, like film directors attempting get the best 'take' or view.

Greg, for example, was an 18-year-old who presented with paedophilic fantasies about young girls. He prided himself on never needing the Internet or risking getting in trouble. Instead, he constantly observed his immediate environment with the intent of looking at, talking to and being nice to the girls he saw. Whilst presenting as caring and benign, he observed from the backroom and seemed to take mental pictures and clips of interactions. Later, when alone, he peeled off the mask and engaged in 'mental photo-shoping', as he called it, imposing his perverse fantasies onto the mental images he collected. As an abused child himself, his particular way of coping with his trauma was to re-enact the process of grooming, focusing on the moment of the unmasking – when the abuser presents his real aim to the child. At that moment, when the victim discovers that he is already trapped, lacking both authority and choice to reject the abuser, he triumphs over the situation by taking part.

Greg's fantasy, therefore, sexualized the backroom process and the moment in which the real intent was revealed, when access had been already gained and resistance was no longer psychologically available. Indeed, this young man's fantasies never reached beyond this moment into further sexualization or enactment. Instead, he felt triumphant about being able to 'offend without ever committing a real illegal act'.

Superheroes versus villains

Some patients focus on the omnipotent idea of possessing 'special backroom powers' and often use cartoon superhero metaphors to describe their experiences. In the superhero position, the patient presents as a conflicted character that manages his past trauma and his attraction to darkness by using his powers for the greater good. In the villain position the patient denies all conflict and fragility by a callous and sadistic excited use of his secret strength.

As in typical superhero comics, both superhero and villain are similar in their actual internal experience in the moment of action, as they use their powers excitedly and without feeling. Similarly, both experience backroom power as a dark force – channelling traumatic energies of past terror and loss.

However, they differ in the way the backroom is equilibrated with the rest of the personality and their capacity to hold on to a full narrative of their experience. A villain presentation (or state of mind), similar to Andy, is callous and cold, calculated and criminal. The superhero, on the other hand, is more conflicted, emotionally alive, and carries with him a mixed experience of containment and trauma, loss and/or issues with intimacy. He relies on the backroom for protection rather than for psychic survival as his villain opponent.

Callum, a masculine, secretly gay rugby playing 16 year old who lost his father at a young age, initially presented as very depressed. However, he became lively and animated when describing his superhero identity in his mission to rescue young women from being used by guys for sex. In doing so he used his 'powers' to warn them of approaching danger by befriending the would-be perpetrators and exposing their intention. He described himself as a double agent, having full access to the masculine world whilst actually being quite contemptuous of it, often joining in homophobic jokes whilst secretly grandiose and vengeful. Undercover, he could gain access and foil the plans of those who predated on the weakest girls in the group. Callum accumulated mass information that he constantly harvested from every 'boys' dressing room' conversation he participated in, sneakily navigating the topics of discussion so they would lead to the data he was after.

Danny, on the other hand, at 22, was the predator type Callum attempted to protect girls from. After a period in therapy he was able to describe himself as a fraudster who hid at the back of his mind and sneakily prescribed to others what he felt they wanted to hear in order to get closer to them. His attitude was one of 'I can be who ever you want me to be' in order to gain trust and access. He used his capacity to amass information about people in the here-and-now of any relationship whilst always keeping an eye open for other bits of information that could lead to new grooming targets. He spoke about a wish to feel a sense of guilt and responsibility but an inability to do so. Instead, although he could recognize the reality of his actions and aim, he could not override his intense excitement and need to enact. In the moment of action, therefore, any shame or guilt was absent. In the aftermath of a big triumph he had a glimpse of a deeply depressive relational desert, which he would quickly get away from by further enactments and the creation of a dismissive narrative in which responsibility would be avoided.

The antisocial backroom

The antisocial tendency according to Winnicott (1950–55) implies hope. Unlike other actions which might go unnoticed, an antisocial act induces an environmental-social reaction to it. As a result, some attention is called to the child and with it a hope that the child's unmet needs would be noticed and attended to.

I believe that all backrooms are antisocial at their core. However, although the unconscious wish to be discovered exists, many backroom operators feel that they risk psychological annihilation if noticed. As a result, the backroom narcissistic structure converts the wish to be discovered and the need to be attended to by caring adults, into a perverse and gratifying secret excitement of being able to fool others, and survive (much like the boy who fooled his TA).

Once the backroom is in full operation, any antisocial acts are in fact backroom failures, coded messages that if deciphered correctly might lead back to the backroom they originated from. Concerned others who attend to the mistakes without noticing the structure are usually confronted by further excitement and contempt by a sophisticated backroom operator who is accustomed to managing mistakes in order to preserve the secret structure.

Some young adults and older backroom operators come to therapy because they suffer the implications of failing to expose their backroom in a way that got the attention they needed. Instead, they suffer the consequences of not being noticed, feeling depressed, caught in an impossible double life, feeling empty or highly addicted to near death (Joseph, 1982), taking huge risks, creating damage but never able to stop. Many of them experience their first real backroom failures in therapy, when their unconscious has been awoken to the fact that there is still hope of being seen.

The adolescent backroom

The backroom can exist uninterrupted for many years, even a lifetime, especially if it is equilibrated with other parts of the personality and heavily reinforced through material and social success. However, especially in adolescence and early adulthood, it can collapse, at least for a while, create crisis and with it an opportunity for change.

Joshua, for example, was 15 when he was referred after developing a fascination with gory and extreme pornography. In the first assessment session he attended with his mother, he presented as pale, unkempt, lost and unfocused. His mother, on the other hand, had a memorable presence; she wore long denim overalls, yellow sandals and her dyed bright red hair made into a long plait. Although expressing concern about her son, she seemed incongruently jolly, as if strangely excited about discussing her son's difficulties.

Joshua's affect was flat. He looked at his mother after each question he was asked and then pause lightly so his sentence could be seamlessly completed by her.

Any aggression or frustrations were completely absent. Instead, there was a strong sense, typical of many such assessments and presentations, that conflicting emotional experiences had to exist in parallel to each other, carefully separated like toxic explosive substances. If allowed to leak and contaminate each other, a catastrophic explosion would follow. Preventing this explosion, through the prism of the core complex (Glasser, 1979), was Joshua's way to control his mother and protect her from his catastrophic aggression.

When Joshua's use of the backroom started to change in therapy, aggression, separation and independence became viable options. As a result, a cycle of progress and regression emerged; Joshua would retreat to the rear, engineer a backroom failure, expose the structure and induce further intrusions and restrictions imposed by his mother. She would then request an urgent review of treatment and complain aggressively that there was no progress, making the therapist feel tricked by the patient who now secretly enjoyed watching the telling-off session.

Most adolescents who manage to expose the backroom eventually do well in therapy, which will be discussed later in this chapter. However, it is important to state at this stage that adolescents are different because of the availability of powerful developmental process that could be put back on track or ignited before the backroom becomes fully formed and operational. As adolescents become able to take real steps towards separation and real intimacy, the backroom tends to be less prominent and needed

The mind-hacker

Most children do not feel that they need to know the full content of their parents' minds because they are not threatened or feel severely tantalized by being excluded from information. They can therefore trust that their parents are both benign in the way they communicate to them, and able to tolerate their aggression when they are not happy about aspects of their experience.

Future mind hackers do not completely trust the content of their parents' minds and/or are unable to tolerate being excluded. Some might even feel hacked into and controlled by a parent who is trying to trick them into something in order to avoid their frustration or aggression and 'keep them quiet'.

Hacking into such parental minds becomes a psychological solution to managing such experiences. The omnipotent mind-hackers feels that nothing can be kept secret from them, which makes them feel safe and later excited and powerful.

Mind hackers arrive in therapy after years of experience in being hyper-vigilant and secretly aware of ways of getting access, which they have been using, feeling powerful and in control.

Modern technology is perfectly suited to this type of relationship with the world; With smartphones in most pockets, a great deal of human communications is conducted without needing to be present in the same place and at the same time. This is a perfect environment for those who avoid being present in the here-and-now of any relationship. There, behind the screen, backroom operators are able to carefully manipulate and design tailor-made messages that if 'clicked on' provide valuable information and access to the hacker.

Ron, (aged 16), was an actual hacker by night and a computer science student by day. He started as a 'punisher', hacking into school and college as revenge for feeling marginalized and mistreated. This, as he later discovered, was only a stepping-stone to becoming a grooming expert, who prided himself on his capacity to get young boys to send him their naked pictures online. Similar to other backroom operators, he sexualized the moment of triumph – getting the picture – rather than use the image he was provided. Like Andy, he felt empowered by knowing that he got someone to act in a way they would have never initiated themselves. However, unlike Andy, Ron oscillated between states of omnipotent excitement, and a depressed state in which he felt ashamed and guilty. The cycle he was caught up in was obviously addictive.

Both Andy and Ron were successful groomers and indeed, grooming is a form of mind-hacking; a groomer hacks into a relationship or creates one with a secret 'backdoor' – open for the hacker to enter as he pleases. With actual intentions hidden from view, the groomer gains access into the victim and suspends their capacity to say no. 'Consent' as it is perceived in this hacked-into relationship is the absence of a no rather than the presence of a yes, passive acceptance rather than an active choice. As mentioned above, it is often the point in which backroom omnipotence is at its highest, sometimes without the need to be followed by an actual enactment to serve as a trophy for the successful hacker/groomer.

The backroom as a forensic enactment

The backroom is the seat of constant enactment, not thoughtful reflection. As such, most backroom patients could be defined as mental offenders in the same way some hackers are able to commit robbery without leaving their desk and without anyone noticing that something had gone missing.

As mentioned earlier, backroom patients use the Internet and social media in order to hack into, groom and control. Equally, they will definitely Google their psychotherapist's name before the first session and alongside the initial stages of therapy. They are likely to dig as deeply as possible using all their IT skills. They are also prone to hold on to any information for further use or be narcissistically enraged if no valuable personal information was available. Similarly, they would scan the consulting room and psychotherapist in detail, be extremely sensitive to any change but might not share this information at all, storing and voyeuristically enjoy peeking without being seen.

As with all forensic patients, enactment in the consulting room is present from the beginning. Avoiding it completely is a highly paradoxical activity with backroom patients because it sends the therapist into a battle of minds with the patient, each trying to avoid being hacked into. Both the hacker-patient and the antivirus-psychotherapist-expert become masters of the same skills which they use against each other. Their dance can be interesting and challenging but never to be mistaken for therapy.

Spotting and working with backroom deception

It might be helpful to start by borrowing Glasser's (1964) differentiation between self-preservative and sadistic violence, and applying it to distinguish between self-preservative and manipulative deception (I'm not using sadistic here in order to keep a wider spectrum).

Almost all the deceptive narratives I have heard from non-backroom patients included an element of self-deception, in which I was invited to listen to the story the patient told himself rather than being overtly lied to or tricked. Other patients consciously lied but did so in order to get away from the consequences of their actions or the expectation to discuss it. I think that all these patients used deception to preserve the self, either protect it from the truth or protect it from the external consequences of the truth being known. Their deception was mostly situational even when conscious, designed to survive a moment rather than an overall relational strategy developed over many years.

Backroom patients, on the other hand, use deception in a manipulative conscious way in order to control a relationship. The actual results of a successful manipulation are usually only secondary to the backroom thrill and sense of power it provides. Obviously there is a self-preservative aspect even to the backroom, especially in some of the cases I described here, where the backroom was a solution to overwhelming core complex anxieties. Backroom manipulation was a way of getting away from the object and controlling it, regulating both the fear of engulfment and the anxiety of aggressively destroying the object.

However, as with other infantile solutions to core complex anxieties, the backroom became a central feature in the way my patients related to anyone, providing addictive excitement, a sense of power and control.

Clinically, therefore, it is very important not to confuse backroom deception with self-preservative deceptive manoeuvres. Self-preservative deceptors might need to be allowed to take their time by a psychotherapist who helps them take the plunge. Those who hide the backroom, on the other hand, and might camouflage it behind a wall of pseudo-self-deception, need a firm hand that does not collude and exposes the deceptive aim and organization.

Spotting the backroom

There is no technique to make the backroom visible. I stumbled across most backrooms by chance, usually when I said something that surprised the backroom and created an atmosphere in which the hidden operator felt almost compelled to step out from the dim backstage and describe his specific talents for the first time.

I asked a young patient recently, still in his first session, to present himself and the problem he was seeking help for. This was a private referral and I had very little knowledge of the boy and his problem. In response he said that he was very emotionally aware and felt that this sensitivity allowed him to make contact with others, understand and help them. I asked what it was that he was actually doing with other people who needed help and he said that he spent many hours giving advice and consult. Most of this activity happened at night, on the phone, in his basement bedroom, whilst his parents were sleeping. He was later too tired to wake on time and hardly made it to school. He said that although he got in trouble with the adults he could not stop because people depended on him.

This boy's backroom deception was exposed when I asked him *how* he helped all those people. I believe that this question surprised the backroom and created a huge temptation to finally come out and expose the great powers of data collection and mind manipulation.

Like many others before him this patient smiled first, and then, over some time, described how having sensitivities allowed him to notice others' fragilities and needs and use those as openings through which he could hack into and get them to feel that he was the only one who could understand. He enjoyed their dependency but more than that – the fantasy that he was already an adult, wise and experienced, not one of many or dependant on teachers and parents, needed to be understood, to be part of a group, do well and slowly develop.

There is no sure way to surprising the backroom apart for being alert to its possible existence in certain cases. It is important to remain flexible, remember that deception is a relationship that has meaning, and not shy away from bold investigation.

Being straightforward

Although all patients are curious about the way their psychotherapists think about them, backroom patient usually believe that psychotherapy is a backroom pursuit. It is therefore crucially important to be very straightforward so the patient is not a recipient of carefully phrased interpretations wisely cooked up in the therapist's mind without the patient noticing.

This means in practice that I try to give the patient an immediate experience of being in the company of someone who shares with them what he thinks rather than passively accumulate information for further therapeutic use. In doing so I explicitly refuse the invitation for participating in a mind-game. I might even address this directly if clinically appropriate and state as I once did, 'I tell you what I think rather than hide my thoughts and prescribe them to you according to a secret therapeutic plan'. I might add, 'If you look for a secret plan you might risk missing the meaning of what I actually say'.

I completely avoid phrasing interpretations in a way that might make patients feel secretly observed, such as 'you are letting me know that...' or 'you might be wondering what I feel / think in relation to...'. These might be helpful tentative comments to patients who unconsciously hide but not those who actively conceal aspects of themselves. Instead, I comment directly about the backroom, voice my concerns about potentially walking into traps or being led, and ask the patient to join me in thinking about the way he is communicating with me and others.

Difficult to treat backroom patients

Most backroom patients who are referred because something they did got exposed, are quick to show their backroom. However, patients presenting as suffering with depression, emptiness or addiction, for example, might find it difficult to step out of hiding. Those patients attempt to have therapy without being completely present. Unlike the patients I presented above, they do not respond to the invitation to share their methods of operation or other deceptive tricks.

The only way to notice their backroom and help them relate more truthfully is to notice what they do with my comments and interpretations when they hear them, and later after leaving the sessions. I once asked a patient, 'are you making direct in-the-moment contact with me or do you use the sessions as a takeaway service, store my comments, and feed yourself elsewhere?'. This type of dynamic is always important to keep in mind anyway, because even the honestly communicating backroom patients might still be storing and sorting interpretations rather than be present, especially if the situation is emotionally demanding.

Although most patients eventually reveal themselves, there is a distinct group of patients who never acknowledge the backroom and remain deceitful and omnipotent. They are usually mental hackers and groomers who arrive to therapy when they realize that they are in psychological trouble but cannot afford to be totally seen because they fear the actual repercussions of past and present activities.

In an attempt to resolve this conflict they hack into therapy like a double agent attempting to gain access to a rival spy-network. First they provide enough genuine information that allows them access to the psychotherapist's thinking mind. Then they steal the comments and interpretations they receive, and use it on themselves internally, unpacking and generalizing it to secretly address what they would never say in the sessions. Unlike the takeaway-service patients, who are psychologically defensive but later develop a capacity to 'eat in', these backroom double agents never really become fully engaged.

The impact of therapy on the backroom

Interestingly, quite a few backroom patients were surprised to find out that they had an unconscious – a part of their mind that they were not in direct control of. They believed that being able to hide so well from others meant that they were totally exposed to themselves. Being able to notice that there is still an unknown part at the core of the way they relate opens the possibility to further therapeutic investigation.

Once the backroom is exposed, patients gain very quick insight into the way they have been relating to others. After a period of sharing their omnipotent backroom powers for the first time, they start noticing gaps in experience and potential unmet needs. Depending on the specific backroom culture, they might notice how the absence of aggression or of intimacy is compensated by hacking and control. Impotent rage is felt when things do not work to plan or if there is a whiff of potential exposure or humiliation. The relational story becomes more complicated, to include aspects of the patient's life that the patient thinks about for the first time in therapy.

Interestingly, I found that backroom patients do not respond well to narrative type interpretations in which their present is explained by their early relational past. Even if the interpretations are appropriately placed in time and in content, they fit a picture of how psychotherapy works and evoke both hacking anxieties and excitements. Instead of attending to the comment emotionally and in a reflective way, many patients seem to pounce on the interpretation as representing something about the way the psychotherapist thinks, try to hack in or just empty the interaction from its meaning.

It is obviously crucial to know the relational past and make links between that and the present. However, I do so by keeping it in mind whilst concentrating on the way patients relate in the here and now of their current lives. At times, especially at the beginning, it feels as if the patient and I inspect interactions frame by frame to spot backroom activity and excitement. Later, as the work expands patients might themselves relate to their past but without delving into the narrative, which seems to suffice.

As patients notice that they are missing out on aspects of life or development, the backroom becomes more of a hindrance than a facilitator. It is then slowly relegated from a glorified control centre to a bleak addicts' den, protecting patients from what they can now see as absence of being emotionally present, intimate or appropriately aggressive. Patients experience more psychic pain and notice real damage inflicted on their relationships now and in the past.

Adolescent patients are often able to start realistically to contemplate separation from parents and a move to an adolescent group that becomes more available. Older patients who live various versions of double lives are either able to move to their first life, letting go of the second, or are recovering in the aftermath of both first and second life collapsing into each other. Either way, the need for the backroom is greatly diminished.

References

Alvarez, A. (2012) *The thinking heart: three levels of psychoanalytic therapy with disturbed children*. London and New York, Routledge.

Campbell, D. (1994) Breaching the shame shield: thoughts on the assessment of adolescent child sexual abusers. *Journal of Child Psychotherapy*. 20, 309–326.

Glasser, M. (1964) Aggression and sadism in perversions. In: Rosen, I. (ed.) *Sexual deviation*. Oxford, Oxford University Press. pp. 279–300.

Glasser, M. (1979) Some aspects of the role of aggression in the perversions. In: Rosen, I. (ed.) *Sexual deviations*. 2nd ed. Oxford, Oxford University Press. pp. 278–305.

Meltzer, D. (1992) *The claustrum. An investigation of claustrophobic phenomena.* Strath Tay, Perth, Clunie Press.

Winnicott, D.W. (1950–55) Aggression in relation to emotional development. In: *Collected papers: through paediatrics to psychoanalysis*. London, Hogarth Press 1975.

Chapter 7

Angels and devils: sadism and violence in children

Graham Music

In this paper, I describe some typical features of violence and sadism in children seen at the Portman Clinic, using the related vertices of psycho-analysis and developmental science. Unsurprisingly, children's violence stirs up strong feelings, and as Alvarez makes clear, 'staring evil in the eye' (Alvarez, 1995) without shirking from its reality requires courage as we generally want to believe the best of our patients. Indeed, many professionals are invested in seeing children as 'angels', clinging to a belief in their hopeful, positive natures, often with a naïve conviction that showing kindness and love is enough, in effect turning a blind eye to what can be too disturbing to face. Others though see such children as innately aggressive and destructive, almost as evil incarnate, with no redeeming features. One of our tasks is to steer a course between the Scylla and Charybdis of these views.

An extreme case is the infamous murderer Mary Bell. Before her 11th birthday she had strangled a four-year-old boy in a derelict house and then strangled a three-year-old in local wasteland, scratched his body and mutilated his penis. In part such behaviour was a re-enactment of her experiences, as she was a victim of hatred, torture and sadism. As clinicians we need to understand both the abusing and abused, both victim and perpetrator in the same person.

To do this work well, we first must manage our own horror. Jamie Bulger, murdered by ten year olds Jon Venables and Robert Thompson, had paint thrown in his eyes, was kicked, stamped on, had bricks thrown at him, an iron bar dropped on him, batteries reportedly pushed into his anus, he had 10 skull fractures and 43 major injuries. Faced with such facts, it is hard to imagine feeling anything but horror and antipathy for the perpetrators. However, they too were victims (c.f. Morrison, 2011) who needed help.

Many Portman referrals arrive due to anxiety in the system about a child, and can feel like hot potatoes that no-one wants to touch, especially if the violence is of a sexual nature. A typical recent example was 8-year-old Bill who had been caught indulging in sexual play in toilets with younger children. Some staff felt he should be excluded from school permanently to safeguard other children, seeing him as already a callous and serial sex offender. Others were fond of him, felt sad about his life experiences and saw him as an innocent victim. He was living with his aunt, after child protection proceedings. His mother had been a drug user who almost certainly prostituted herself and his father was probably his mother's pimp. He had been coming to school unkempt and dirty, but this had improved since living with his aunt.

Bill's case raises many common dilemmas. He could be aggressive and cruel, had few friends and enjoyed hurting other children. This had abated somewhat in recent months and it was not clear why. Was this cruelty a way of getting rid of his own bad feelings, a classic form of projection? Was the lessening of his aggression a sign of feeling due to better care? Or was he just becoming more sophisticated in his manipulations? Was his aggression mainly cold and calculated or more a reactive response to frustration? Should the positive and caring feelings he evoked in adults be trusted? For example, he enjoyed the attention of his Learning Support Assistant and often snuggled into her. Was this a form of manipulative overly sexualized contact masquerading as innocent affection-seeking? Such questions often need unpicking in making sense of such children. In what follows I introduce a few key themes central to understanding this patient group, using brief vignettes.

A core Portman concept, the core complex

Glasser's concept of the core complex which has similarities to what is sometimes described as the claustro-agorphobic syndrome or shuttle (Rey & Magagna, 1994), is seen commonly in sadistic and aggressive patients and in perversions (Glasser, 1986, 1992) where patients can bear neither closeness nor separation from the object. Glasser saw the core complex as a universal stage that all must go through, but I prefer to see it as a compromise formation in response to difficult early experiences. For Glasser the core complex provides a solution to these issues, often in the form of addiction to a sexual or aggressive act.

A 17-year-old Georgio was already addicted to sadomasochistic fetishistic sexual encounters. These allowed a degree of closeness and contact, avoiding the awful desolation of aloneness and separation from the object but without the need for actual intimacy. In Georgios's case this made sense in terms of him having a very intrusive mother and violent father. His fetish and accompanying fantasies recapitulated some of his early traumatic experiences and he also sought out pornography which contained both the sadomasochistic and fetishistic elements, fuelling this fantasy.

Typically, Georgio's core complex was marked by withdrawal from the object, from a fear of being engulfed, leading to an unbearable dread and aloneness which in turn led to clinging to the object, a need to take control and possession of it, sometimes violently. A narcissistic and omnipotent psychic organization can result, in which power and control is relied upon, often sexual power, rather than real object relating. Loneliness and abandonment are avoided via aggression and control, often sexualized. In this solution to the core complex, both proximity and distance are retained via the aggressive or perverse sexual act. However, the cost is that any hope for real object relating gets lost as there is a disavowal of real love and care from another, much as seen in what Rosenfeld describes as narcissistic defences (Rosenfeld, 1987). The painfulness of beginning to bear such feelings of emotional contact with, and separation from, the object often becomes central to therapeutic work, particularly in the transference.

Aggression, cold and hot kinds

Presentations of anti-social tendencies with the core complex issues at their core can arise as a compromise when early experiences of emotional safety are lacking. Most of our sadistic or aggressive patients have witnessed both trauma and neglect in early childhood but, equally importantly, have missed out on good enough early experiences which allow, as Winnicott suggested (1954), an easeful going-on-being from which the psyche can begin to reside in the soma safely. The violent perpetrators we work with have mostly both endured horrendous early experiences, and lacked hope and trust-inducing human relationships. Thus they often resort to core-complex solutions to unbearable feelings, in the form of violence, sadism or sexual fetishism.

Some children commit sadistic acts in the heat of the moment and are best understood as displaying an impulsive 'hot-blooded' kind of aggression. They feel upset, provoked and want to hurt back, often because something feels 'unfair'. This is different to 'colder' more proactive kinds of aggression, in which children and adults show more calculation. Proactive aggressors do not feel bad about their anger, whereas impulsive reactive types often do (Arsenio et al., 2009).

Such impulsivity and an inability to tolerate frustration, often fuelled by early trauma, can lead to a quickly triggered threat system, leading to aggression and a wish to hurt others. Such people often have poor social skills and misread cues, perhaps seeing anger or contempt where others would not. This can be a variant of self-preservative aggression (Yakeley, 2009), in which the other is seen as a serious, even life-threatening, threat. A sense of being easily shamed is also common in such cases, often leading to swift reactivity.

Children who suffer violence and trauma often lack much empathy and mentalizing capacity, believing that life is not fair, safe or reliable. More reactive children and adults often seek justice but they misperceive the motivations of others and can very easily feel that they are 'victims'. Their physiological arousal, such as heart-rate, shallow breathing or sweating, tends to be greater (Hubbard et al., 2010), their amygdala firing more strongly than the average person in response to pictures containing violence or threat (Qiao et al., 2012). Reactive aggression is associated with lower attention spans, worse verbal ability and high autonomic reactivity (McLaughlin et al., 2014). We need to feel relatively safe and calm in order for the brain regions central to empathy and compassion to be online (Gilbert, 2009) but it makes no sense to feel calm, empathic or reflective when living a life that feels full of threat and danger.

A typical case: Shane

Shane, six, had a background of serious abuse and neglect, was in foster care, and capable of great cruelty. His mother had been a drug-addicted victim of domestic violence, much of which he had witnessed, abandoning him at aged two, after which he had seven foster placements.

He was violent with other children, had few friends, struggling to control himself, concentrate or learn. In my assessment, I felt an edge of threat from him, finding that I was breathing shallowly, bracing for something scary to happen. I find I rely increasingly on my embodied countertransference with such patients.

Shane stated that the toys in the box were 'for girls', a sign of his fear of softness and vulnerability as well as his lack of capacity for symbolic play. In games he was always determined to win, and then would yelp triumphantly and look disdainfully in me. He often left me feeling tricked, betrayed and stupid, clearly projecting something of his own cruel experience into me. He had enough understanding of my thoughts and feelings to work out how to trick me, but this was very different from empathy. I did though feel that Shane's coldness was defensive, not primary, he conveyed a fear of closeness, but also some hope for it, in classic core-complex style.

For children like Shane, often the work is at a very basic level, such as naming emotions, but with feeling ('that made you very, very angry'). He was in identification with ruthless alpha-male idols and resisted contact with softer kinder aspects of his personality. It was crucial that I bore and accepted his identification with aggressive cruel figures. As Eigen (1975) suggested, sometimes antisocial tendencies need to be tolerated, even accepted by us, as the libidinous expression of such urges can then be utilized for the sake of 'deep personality repair and development'. This cannot happen if we refuse to bear such cruelty with our patients.

In response to Shane's poor symbolic capacity I began playing with toy animals in front of him. Soon I he began to play himself and I witnessed a series of killings of large and small toy animals, undertaken gleefully and triumphantly. Chilling as this was, it allowed me to talk about feelings and what was happening, acknowledging with as little judgement as I could muster, his pleasure in the sadistic attacks. This in turn enabled him to continue playing.

Tiny moments of hope crept in. In one session mid-game he momentarily hesitated. Normally, I would have missed the moment but this time I asked where his mind was. He looked surprised and then said 'I was thinking about Miss Smith' (his former teacher), such flickering self-awareness hopefully a sign of the tiniest beginnings of a thinker who could think thoughts (Bion, 1962). I simply said 'wow Shane you really are having thoughts, a person who can think things'. This led to him saying how he wished he was still at his old school and how 'I think about it lots of time'.

His progress depended not just on me bearing the negative but also building the positive. The end of his pencil kept breaking, something that would have made him very angry previously, but this time he said 'ok I can do it' as he determinedly sharpened it, building on his experience of my belief in him and that things could come right.

The months that followed saw further shifts. He would pause for a moment as if listening or thinking. He could not say what he was thinking at first, but he liked it when I acknowledged his mind growing. In time small half thoughts crept into the room, and eventually memories, such as of earlier benign figures. As the months went on I noticed him being interested in me, listening to me, watching my expressions, and even beginning to help me to put away his things into the box. Similar changes were being spotted at home and school.

Shane never became the calmest or most loving boy, but he started to change. As he began to develop some belief that the world could be safe, and that some people such as his carer could be trusted, something had begun to soften in him. Shane's sadism had been primarily projective and defensive and lessened when he felt safe enough. It reared its head still when he felt threat but new personality traits were forming, kinder internal objects, more benign brain pathways and softer bodily systems that could be accessed when he felt safe enough.

Cold aggressors

Unlike Shane, some children show a colder, more proactive form of aggression, targeting others to achieve definite goals for themselves. They might read minds and intentions well but have little fellow-feeling or empathy. Those who display proactive aggression often do so in a calculated way and have sometimes been described as 'happy victimisers' (Smith et al., 2010) but can also respond reactively when they feel angry (Thornton et al., 2013).

Unlike the reactive children who often cry out against unfairness, cold-hearted aggressors care little about those they harm, lacking remorse (Arsenio & Lemerise, 2010). Colder forms of aggression are harder to treat, partly because perpetrators often have less desire to change, and are motivated by gains from being aggressive.

As Arsenio and Gold suggests (2006), those coming from backgrounds where love, support and empathy were not available, can believe that relationships are about power, control, and domination. Many display severe anti-social tendencies, impulsivity and behavioural problems, sometimes labelled as having *callous-unemotional* traits (Viding et al., 2008), and such traits come with a poor prognosis (Frick & White, 2008).

Many adult psychopaths were anti-social children, started fires, torturing pets and showing cruelty. The presence of callous-unemotional traits in children, alongside conduct disorders, hugely increases the likelihood of serious offending, violent crime and shorter periods between re-offending (Brandt et al., 1997). Their cold-heartedness seems more than a metaphor, as low heart-rates is predictive of classic callous-unemotional traits like lying and fearlessness, (Dierckx et al., 2014), low autonomic arousal and fearlessness being predictive of later behavioural problems (Baker et al., 2013).

Unlike impulsively aggressive children, those with callous-unemotional traits barely react to negative cues, for example showing minimal amygdala responses in the face of fear (Jones et al., 2009), and low physiological arousal, for example less sweating or fast breathing, when shown pictures of violence or horrific injuries. Often the lower the reactivity in brain areas that register another's pain the worse the psychopathic traits (Marsh et al., 2013), while prefrontal areas necessary for empathy are also less activated (Decety J, 2013). Many abused children I work with show high levels of fearlessness alongside impulsive traits, maybe stealing or hurting others on a whim.

Twelve-year-old Mick was adopted at four from a substance-misusing neglectful and promiscuous mother and a violent father and was probably abused by a paedophile ring, He was excluded on his first week at school, had a tough, steely side to him, his interactions with others were instrumental, based on what he could get, and he took pleasure in seeing others in pain. In his play dolls were mutilated and tortured to his evident enjoyment. While he was hypervigilant enough to monitor me and others for signs of danger, he showed no interest in other people's minds and feelings, except to use for his own ends. I often felt chilled in his presence and a dread of seeing him.

It seemed unlikely that before adoption anyone would have shown interest in his thoughts or feelings. He was particularly cruel to his little sister. When I mentioned her in a session his eyes went icy cold, and at home his parents reported finding him twisting her arm right back, squeezing her as hard as he could, showing no remorse when he hurt her.

Typically, in one early session, he told me smirking that he had deliberately kicked a child in the chest and broken several ribs. Therapeutically it was important to show him that I could bear and tolerate the depth of his cruelty, but not condone it. Ironically, he described his violence as 'therapy', because it made him feel better, telling me how he feels better if he gets revenge. He talked about how you need to get back at people, saying 'I have no choice'. I questioned this, and he insisted that it was their fault, clearly living in Klein's paranoid-schizoid position (Klein, 1946) with an unshakeable conviction in the law of talion.

Just as Alvarez (1992) and others have argued that, when working with autistic children, we have to find and help to grow the 'non-autistic' parts of the personality, with callous-unemotional children like Mick we have to try and find and make a relationship with non-callous more hopeful aspects of the personality, however small and fragile, without being naïve Pollyanna-ish.

After quite some time, there was the slightest hint that Mick was starting to acknowledge some neediness and upset. He had struggled with a break during which he was particularly unhappy but also nasty to those around him. He could not acknowledge any dependence on me until I forcefully said, in therapist-centred style, how I felt sad that he had lost any idea that he as in my mind over the break. He looked sad, albeit just momentarily, and then squirmed out of this feeling. I said that he was determined that we would not leave here without me really feeling something of how desperate he felt and he asked 'well do you?', with sadistic pleasure I thought. I struggled, as often, with whether there was anything hopeful here, perhaps at best a desire to be understood via projecting feelings. It is easy to feel either too hopeless or falsely hopeful with such patients.

In the end my therapy with Mick was not the most successful, in part because his foster placement broke down and he had to leave the area. Placements of children with callous traits often fail, not surprisingly; they are hard to like and warm to. Progress had been slow anyway, and he had continued to remorselessly bully other children, manipulate and show little concern. He left just as some soft edges were beginning to come through and I will never know if these could have been built upon.

Mick, typically, was on course for gaining a criminal record and had already been found stealing, bullying, causing serious injury and damage to property. We are not sure why some children experiencing terrible neglect and abuse are more likely to develop in this way than others. Viding (Viding et al., 2012) and colleagues have suggested a genetic component. However it is almost unheard of to come across a violent or psychopathic criminal having a relatively ordinary childhood, and often the stories are unthinkably horrendous (Gullhaugen & Nøttestad, 2011, 2012). Indeed, any visit to a high security prison reveals consistent tales of adults with early lives marked by trauma and lack of basic parenting.

Poor early attachment (Pasalich et al., 2012), maltreatment (Kimonis et al., 2013) and neglect (Kumsta et al., 2012) are linked to callous-unemotional traits. Several studies have found links between early trauma and psychopathy (Patrick et al., 2010; Poythress et al., 2006). I have suggested that it is either neglect, the absence of good experiences, and/or dissociative processes, which lead to the kind of dampened down lack of reactivity we see in psychopath, even if neglect can be harder to spot (Music, 2009). These are extremely tough patients to treat. Adult psychopaths rarely present for treatment and callous-unemotional children are rarely worried about themselves, even if adults around them are.

Addiction and sexual sadism

In many patients, we see addictive and sometimes sexual excitement in inflicting pain (Bower et al., 2012). Much addictive behaviour starts for defensive reasons, perhaps as attempts to manage core complex anxieties, stress, trauma or feelings of inadequacy. However, such defences often themselves become addictive in similar ways to gambling, drugs or pornography. Typical is how many soldiers in war-torn areas speak of the excitement of fighting and killing (Weierstall et al., 2013), many returning to warzones because fighting again warded off post-traumatic stress symptoms (Weierstall et al., 2012).

Many children and adults take pleasure in another's suffering, probably a distortion of ordinary *schadenfreude*, in which clear reward circuits in the brain fire up and empathic brain circuitry gets turned off (Bhanji & Delgado, 2014). To perpetrate aggression fellow-feeling for the victim must be obliterated, requiring a narcissistic, non-object-related state of mind. As Meloy and Shiva (2007) has shown, in the psychopath we not only see low levels of anxiety and fear, but also a severely constricted affective world, poor emotional literacy, and capacities for object relating. Meloy suggests that they tend to function at a pre-oedipal level, with little capacity for identification or internalization, or anything that might resemble a superego. They often identify with their aggressors though, in the sense that Anna Freud described (Freud, 1972), in part to deny and project shame and humiliation.

Perhaps partly because of such a poorly developed internal and emotional worlds, such perpetrators often experience a form of psychic deadness, as Gilligan and others have shown (Gilligan, 2009). It is no coincidence that patients at the Portman clinic often re-offend at times of emotional stress or pain. Such patients struggle to process feelings and their sexual violence and aggression can become a kind of compensatory addictive antidepressant. As Nathanson writes (this volume) pressing the 'fuck-it button' gives rise to a triumphant thrill.

Eleven-year-old Les was caught forcing his nine-year-old brother to suck his penis. There was a long intergenerational history of sexual abuse and violence. Relationships in this family were based on fear and asserting power. On our advice social services removed Les and he was placed in a residential unit. Here though he continued to be a risk to other children, particularly when something happened which would stir up difficult feelings, such as his key-worker being away. Les had poor emotional vocabulary, little trust and treated most people with contempt. In therapy sessions he was another who loved to trick me and then smirk with disdainful pleasure. We learnt not only about terrible violence towards his mother from her partners, but also historical acts perpetrated by Les himself, including molesting a very young child. Les seemed almost uncontrollably driven to act in this way. Given any access to the internet he would watch pornography.

Yet as I got to know him I was struck by the paucity of his internal world and mind, which seemed empty and flat. It became apparent that the recourse to sexual stimulation, often at others' expense, was a way of feeling less dead. Until healthier ways of feeling real and emotionally alive could be developed he would continue to behave as he did.

Sadistic sexual acts such as those perpetrated by Les, are perhaps the ones that stir up the biggest anxieties in professionals. Many have been victims of sexual offences themselves (Ogloff et al., 2012), and come from backgrounds high in conflict, neglect and poor emotional care (Riser et al., 2013). The lack of experiences of empathy and care, alongside overt cruelty, can lead to excitement and pleasure in aggressive and sexual acts. Such children and young people tend to have a view of the world, and of other people, as fundamentally untrustworthy and dangerous (De Ganck & Vanheule, 2015).

In adolescence, when the dopaminergic circuitry is fast developing (Blakemore & Mills, 2014), risks of addictive behaviours are heightened, whether to drugs, computer games or sexual and other forms of cruelty and sadism. Often what starts as an understandable defence, such as hurting another because one is feeling hurt oneself, can transform into a behaviour which becomes pleasurable in its own right, and addictively so.

It is a tough challenge to know when to hold onto hope and when to focus unflinchingly at what seems like evil, and this certainly requires facing up to the reality of the pleasures and gains perpetrators receive from such addictive sadistic pleasure. In Les' case therapy was not enough, he made small inroads at best, although these increased somewhat after careful work was done with the system and network. This included ongoing consultation to professionals around him, both about boundary setting and about the depth of the dangers he posed to others. Therapy can be offered too early with young people like Les, and instead holding and containing the system must be the first step. Les is one of many cases where therapy ended, seemingly prematurely, but interestingly he reappeared nearly a year later after the system around him had been consolidated.

Sophia: a case of aggression with core complex elements

Sophia's case provides a more hopeful example. Her presentation included many typical Portman presenting issues. She took sadistic pleasure in her aggression, was filled up with core complex anxieties, addicted to sexual and other forms of power. At first at least it was hard to decipher the extent to which her aggression was callous or reactive.

She was 17 when referred following violence and aggressive sexual enactments. I was struck by her tall angular gait, her tough 'masculine' stance and threatening posture. She talked about hitting her boyfriend regularly, was disparaging of any weak or vulnerable feelings, and immediately stated that she would never admit if she cared for someone.

Sophia had good reason to defend the soft aspects of herself. She had experienced the early trauma of long-term hospitalizations, and had older tough and macho brothers who would tease and taunt her. She had to develop effective armour and weaponry, especially as she had never had a parental figure with whom to express a sad, or soft side.

Sophie had a proclivity for aggressive and often violent sexual encounters wherever, whenever and with whomever the temptation arose in her. These acts were a confusing mixture of a wish for intimacy, and a callous attack on dependency needs, and led her to treat others as there to satisfy her needs

Not surprisingly in the transference I too was a potential 'conquest'. In the second month she came into a session flirtatiously, asking me if I liked her clothes, telling me that she spends most of the day nearly naked (working as a swimming coach), letting me know of sexual encounters, and speaking of how she fancied older unshaven men who were mysterious. I felt like potential prey.

In time I saw glimpses of something softer in her which grew as therapy proceeded, such as mentioning her sympathy for a two-year-old cousin who she witnessed being bullied. She was able to wonder if she was a wanted baby, whether her parents had ever loved each other, in other words whether a loving sexual encounter was possible. She talked about her shame of her scars that remained from her early operations, something she needed to keep hidden, and of course I thought about her being even more wary of exposing her raw emotional wounds. She was able to admit how scared she was of the night, of being alone, and in time dared to think about the possibility of a real relationship. Whenever she neared such vulnerability I witnessed a backlash and she attacked any softness, in herself and others. If I showed sympathy for this soft side of her or others I too was dumped into the category of the soft and useless, her highly armoured carapace (Bion, 1986), guarding powerfully against the dangers of vulnerability.

If I talked about her fear of her own vulnerability she thought that I was joining the side of strength against weakness (hers). If I talked about my need to tolerate softer aspects of her, she felt, to start with at least, that I was speaking from a position of smug superiority, and interpretations made from a more distant place seemed to give me, in her eyes, a steely aura, one she was too impressed by.

One week she explained, rather nonchalantly that she had had a fight with her new partner, and had-become violent. Yet this time, unusually, she could let me know that she felt let down and hurt, feelings she could not previously have acknowledged.

She developed a fascination for my previous patient, who would often leave crying, Sophia describing this as akin to the strange behaviours of an alien from outer space, suggesting that. this patient was pathetic. Over time she began to ask about the tissues in the room (what they were there for? who might use them? why did I put them there?} and slowly they changed in her mind from weapons of torture to something else. Mostly such tentative moves towards vulnerability were swiftly followed by a harsh re-emergence of her most vicious side, but real change was happening.

She began to report dreams which now had meaning, and had in them loving figures, no longer just constant nightmares of violence and hatred. She reported that her new partner had said 'I love you', and Sophie begrudgingly admitted to me that she liked this. She badly needed me to help her bear such soft feelings, rather than rubbish them, and in such moments, I talked both firmly and from the heart about these changes. Without the firmness in my voice I was ridiculed and denigrated as soft and impotent; yet without the 'heartfelt' and softer tone in my voice, I had little impact. In time this had an effect, stirring something to life, allowing a long buried seed to begin to grow.

About a year in she was actually able to say, in response to an interpretation from me, 'I want to have the loving feelings, but it is best to be a bastard and hurt others'. The harshness was still needed to protect the fledgling softness. She told me, bravely about her feelings following an abortion a few years before. It was another 6 months before the tiniest hint of tears arrived but gentleness was taking root, softening things up inside.

After 18 months she was preparing to leave to go to College. An ending was looming. She asked what would happen with a tear in her eye, and talked about not liking change, how she has kept her own dentist and doctor for a long time. She started to wonder about my life; am I married? She became flirtatious again, I thought attacking the safety and trust we had achieved. She told me about an older teacher she had seduced. I talked of how it might be easier to destroy what we had gained than face the pain of ending, but that she needed to trust that I could bear with her the pain of being in touch with such excruciating feelings. She heard this differently now, with a definite hint of relief, gratitude.

She seemed to soften, even in her body, becoming more feminine; changing the kind of clothes she wore, sporting a fringe, and becoming less brash and harsh in her gestures. Harshness could creep back, but was not so strong any longer, maybe rather like a protective parent who at last feels that its progeny is nearer being able to fend for itself. As we neared our ending, we spent more time thinking about her painful and traumatic childhood, mourning what she did not have.

She could now take in something more helpful and nourishing, becoming able to receive empathic comments from me which previously would have been met with disdain. She was forming a few better friendships and was in a more trusting relationship, allowing herself to be somewhat dependent. Before the final holiday break she was able to describe her wish to retaliate, by leaving therapy prematurely, just as she threatened to be unfaithful in her relationship when her vulnerability was triggered. Core complex issues remained but by the end she could allow herself to stay with her upset and worries, no longer believing that I was enjoying her weakness from a superior place. Alongside the changes in her internal world, and in the way she began to act in the world, I found myself feeling much more warmly towards her in a way that was unthinkable at the start. She could now evoke compassion in others.

Summary

In this paper, I have looked at sadistic behaviour in children and young people, alongside violence, addictive pleasure in aggression and at the different forms of psychic organization seen in reactive and more callous presentations. I have discussed the difficulty of acknowledging real sadism and cruelty in children while holding onto hope. A focus has been how sadistic and aggressive acts can often be defensive, and projective, and attention has been given to the power of core complex anxieties. I have also discussed how behaviours that begin as defences against unbearable psychic experience can become character traits, addictive ones, harnessing the same brain pathways as other forms of addiction. I have suggested that real change is hard to achieve, hard-won, but is certainly possible, more so in more reactive than callous presentations. In such cases, sadism and 'evil' must be looked in the eye while holding onto genuine hope for trusting human relationships.

References

Alvarez, A. (1992) *Live company*. London, Routledge.
Alvarez, A. (1995) Motiveless malignity: problems in the psychotherapy of psychopathic patients. *Journal of Child Psychotherapy*. 21 (2), 167–182.
Arsenio, W. F., Adams, E. & Gold, J. (2009) Social information processing, moral reasoning, and emotion attributions: relations with adolescents' reactive and proactive aggression. *Child Development*. 80 (6), 1739–1755.
Arsenio, W. F. & Gold, J. (2006) The effects of social injustice and inequality on children's moral judgments and behavior: towards a theoretical model. *Cognitive Development*. 21 (4), 388–400.
Arsenio, W. F. & Lemerise, E. A. (eds.) (2010) *Emotions, aggression, and morality in children: bridging development and psychopathology*. Washington, American Psychological Association.
Baker, E., Shelton, K. H., Baibazarova, E., Hay, D. F. & van Goozen, S. H. (2013) Low skin conductance activity in infancy predicts aggression in toddlers 2 years later. *Psychological Science*. 24 (6), 1051–1056.
Bhanji, J. P. & Delgado, M. R. (2014) The social brain and reward: social information processing in the human striatum. *Wiley Interdisciplinary Reviews: Cognitive Science*. 5 (1), 61–73.
Bion, W. R. (1962) A theory of thinking. *Melanie Klein today: developments in theory and practice*. 1, 178–186.

Bion, W. R. (1986) *The long weekend: part of a life.* London, Free Association Books.

Blakemore, S.-J. & Mills, K. L. (2014) Is adolescence a sensitive period for socio-cultural processing? *Annual Review of Psychology.* 65, 187–207.

Bower, M., Hale, R. & Wood, H. (eds.) (2012) *Addictive states of mind.* London, Karnac Books.

Brandt, J. R., Kennedy, W. A., Patrick, C. J. & Curtin, J. J. (1997) Assessment of psychopathy in a population of incarcerated adolescent offenders. *Psychological Assessment.* 9 (4), 429–435.

De Ganck, J. & Vanheule, S. (2015) "Bad boys don't cry": a thematic analysis of interpersonal dynamics in interview narratives of young offenders with psycho-pathic traits. *Frontiers in Psychology.* 6, 960, doi:10.3389/fpsyg.2015.00960. PMID: 26217279; PMCID: PMC4493321.

Decety, J., Skelly, L.R., & Kiehl, K.A. (2013) Brain response to empathy-eliciting scenarios involving pain in incarcerated individuals with psychopathy. *JAMA Psychiatry.* 70(6), 638–645. doi:10.1001/jamapsychiatry.2013.27. PMID: 23615636; PMCID: PMC3914759.

Dierckx, B., Kok, R., Tulen, J. H., Jaddoe, V. W., Hofman, A., Verhulst, F. C., Bakermans-Kranenburg, M. J., Ijzendoorn, M. H. & Tiemeier, H. (2014) A pro-spective study of heart rate and externalising behaviours in young children. *Journal of Child Psychology and Psychiatry.* 55 (4), 402–410.

Eigen, M. (1975) Psychopathy and individuation. *Psychotherapy: Theory, Research & Practice.* 12 (3), 286–294.

Freud, A. (1972) Comments on aggression. *International Journal of Psycho-Analysis.* 53, 163–171.

Frick, P. J. & White, S. F. (2008) Research review: the importance of callous-unemotional traits for developmental models of aggressive and antisocial behavior. *Journal of Child Psychology and Psychiatry.* 49 (4), 359–375.

Gilbert, P. (2009) *The compassionate mind.* London, Constable-Robinson.

Gilligan, J. (2009) Sex, gender and violence: Estela Welldon's contribution to our understanding of the psychopathology of violence. *British Journal of Psychotherapy.* 25 (2), 239–256.

Glasser, M. (1986) Identification and its vicissitudes as observed in the perversions. *The International Journal of Psychoanalysis.* 67 (1), 9–17.

Glasser, M. (1992) Problems in the psychoanalysis of certain narcissistic disorders. *The International Journal of Psychoanalysis.* 73 (3), 493–503.

Gullhaugen, A. S. & Nøttestad, J. A. (2011) Looking for the Hannibal behind the Cannibal: current status of case research. *International Journal of Offender Therapy and Comparative Criminology.* 55 (3), 350–369. doi:10.1177/0306624X10362659

Gullhaugen, A. S. & Nøttestad, J. A. (2012) Under the surface the dynamic inter-personal and affective world of psychopathic high-security and detention pris-oners. *International Journal of Offender Therapy and Comparative Criminology.* 56 (6), 917–936.

Hubbard, J. A., McAuliffe, M. D., Morrow, M. T. & Romano, L. J. (2010) Reactive and proactive aggression in childhood and adolescence: precursors, outcomes, processes, experiences, and measurement. *Journal of Personality.* 78 (1), 95–118.

Jones, A., Laurens, K., Herba, C., Barker, G. & Viding, E. (2009) Amygdala hypoactivity to fearful faces in boys with conduct problems and callous-unemotional traits. *American Journal of Psychiatry*. 166 (1), 95–102.

Kimonis, E. R., Cross, B., Howard, A. & Donoghue, K. (2013) Maternal care, maltreatment and callous-unemotional traits among urban male juvenile offenders. *Journal of Youth and Adolescence*. 42(2), 165–167. doi:10.1007/s10964-012-9820-5. Epub 2012 Sep 30.

Klein, M. (1946) Notes on some schizoid mechanisms. *International Journal of Psycho-Analysis*. 27, 99–110.

Kumsta, R., Sonuga-Barke, E. & Rutter, M. (2012) Adolescent callous–unemotional traits and conduct disorder in adoptees exposed to severe early deprivation. *The British Journal of Psychiatry*. 200 (3), 197–201.

Marsh, A. A., Finger, E. C., Fowler, K. A., Adalio, C. J., Jurkowitz, I. T. N., Schechter, J. C., Pine, D. S., Decety, J. & Blair, R. J. R. (2013) Empathic responsiveness in amygdala and anterior cingulate cortex in youths with psychopathic traits. *Journal of Child Psychology and Psychiatry*. 54(8), 900–910. doi:1 0.1111/jcpp.12063

McLaughlin, K. A., Sheridan, M. A., Alves, S. & Mendes, W. B. (2014) Child maltreatment and autonomic nervous system reactivity: identifying dysregulated stress reactivity patterns by using the biopsychosocial model of challenge and threat. *Psychosomatic Medicine*. 76 (7), 538–546.

Meloy, J. R. & Shiva, A. (2007) A psychoanalytic view of the psychopath. In: Felthous, A. & Sab, H. (eds.) *The international handbook of psychopathic disorders and the law*. Sussex, Wiley. pp. 335–346.

Morrison, B. (2011) *As if*. London, Granta Books.

Music, G. (2009) Neglecting neglect: some thoughts about children who have lacked good input, and are 'undrawn' and 'unenjoyed'. *Journal of Child Psychotherapy*. 35 (2), 142–156.

Ogloff, J. R., Cutajar, M. C., Mann, E., Mullen, P., Wei, F. T. Y., Hassan, H. A. B. & Yih, T. H. (2012) Child sexual abuse and subsequent offending and victimisation: a 45 year follow-up study. *Trends and Issues in Crime and Criminal Justice*. 440 (1), 1836–2206.

Pasalich, D. S., Dadds, M. R., Hawes, D. J. & Brennan, J. (2012) Attachment and callous-unemotional traits in children with early-onset conduct problems. *Journal of Child Psychology and Psychiatry, and Allied Disciplines*. 53 (8), 838–845.

Patrick, C. J., Fowles, D. C. & Krueger, R. F. (2010) Triarchic conceptualization of psychopathy: developmental origins of disinhibition, boldness, and meanness. *Development and Psychopathology*. 21 (3), 913–938.

Poythress, N. G., Skeem, J. L. & Lilienfeld, S. O. (2006) Associations among early abuse, dissociation, and psychopathy in an offender sample. *Journal of Abnormal Psychology*. 115 (2), 288–297. doi:10.1037/0021-843X.115.2.288

Qiao, Y., Xie, B. & Du, X. (2012) Abnormal response to emotional stimulus in male adolescents with violent behavior in China. *European Child & Adolescent Psychiatry*. 21, 193–198.

Rey, H. & Magagna, J. E. (1994) *Universals of psychoanalysis in the treatment of psychotic and borderline states: factors of space-time and language*. London, Free Association Books.

Riser, D. K., Pegram, S. E. & Farley, J. P. (2013) Adolescent and young adult male sex offenders: understanding the role of recidivism. *Journal of Child Sexual Abuse.* 22 (1), 9–31.

Rosenfeld, H. A. (1987) *Impasse and interpretation: therapeutic and anti-therapeutic factors in the psycho-analytic treatment of psychotic, borderline, and neurotic patients.* Oxford, Routledge.

Smith, C. E., Chen, D. & Harris, P. L. (2010) When the happy victimizer says sorry: children's understanding of apology and emotion. *The British Journal of Developmental Psychology.* 28 (Pt 4), 727–746.

Thornton, L. C., Frick, P. J., Crapanzano, A. M. & Terranova, A. M. (2013) The incremental utility of callous-unemotional traits and conduct problems in predicting aggression and bullying in a community sample of boys and girls. *Psychological Assessment.* 25 (2), 366–378. doi:10.1037/a0031153

Viding, E., Fontaine, N. M. & McCrory, E. J. (2012) Antisocial behaviour in children with and without callous-unemotional traits. *Journal of the Royal Society of Medicine.* 105 (5), 195–200.

Viding, E., Jones, A. P., Paul, J. F., Moffitt, T. E. & Plomin, R. (2008) Heritability of antisocial behaviour at 9: do callous-unemotional traits matter? *Developmental Science.* 11 (1), 17–22.

Weierstall, R., Schalinski, I., Crombach, A., Hecker, T. & Elbert, T. (2012) When combat prevents PTSD symptoms—results from a survey with former child soldiers in Northern Uganda. *BMC Psychiatry.* 12 (41), 1–8.

Weierstall, R., Schauer, M. & Elbert, T. (2013) An appetite for aggression. *Scientific American Mind.* 24 (2), 46–49.

Winnicott, D. W. (1954) Mind and its relation to the psyche-soma*. *British Journal of Medical Psychology.* 27 (4), 201–209.

Yakeley, J. (2009) *Working with violence: a contemporary psychoanalytic approach.* London, Palgrave Macmillan.

Chapter 8

Oedipal aspirations and phallic fears: on fetishistic presentation in childhood and young adulthood[1]

Ann Horne

This chapter explores work with a young man who cross-dressed, wore nappies in bed and was preoccupied with pregnant women. When we engage with young people seemingly en route to what once was termed a perverse resolution we encounter early insult, primitive defences and real fear of the oedipal constellation. Within such 'solutions' there can be an element of deception – concealing the phallus to protect it and triumphing over the object in so doing. Technically, it is important to keep a developmental, relational *and* psychosexual framework in mind, to be aware of the subtle invitation to collude with the deception and to maintain close observation of one's counter-transference (Baker, 1994; Carignan, 1999; Renik, 1992).

Stanley

Stanley is an only child. Referred at 19 for psychotherapy following anxiety that he might be paedophilic, he constantly drew mothers, babies and pregnant women, downloaded similar pictures from the internet and videoed mother-and-baby advertisements for baby products. This behaviour had become increasingly obsessive over the past year. He told the referring psychiatrist that he also dressed in women's clothes but now did so rarely. These activities, he maintained, did not give him any sexual arousal. The psychiatrist thought Stanley was not a paedophile but that he could use and needed psychoanalytic psychotherapy.

It emerged that the family's impulse to refer him arose after his mother accepted a new partner, Jim, into the home. Neither Stanley nor his mother had expressed any deep concern prior to this. The presence of a man, and of an oedipal third, was therefore the precipitant. It may also have been the precipitant for increasing his obsessional behaviours. Interestingly, I found myself meeting with Stanley's mother and Jim without Stanley at one point, as I would with a young child. I have reflected on my thoughtlessness, my focus on 'Stanley-the-child' rather than on 'Stanley-the-young-man-of-nearly-20'. It has been vital to retain in mind the strong counter-transference pressure *not* to see Stanley as a potent male – and to recognize behind this his anxieties about being phallic and being perceived to be so.

Stanley was delivered by Caesarean section four weeks prematurely, spending several weeks in an incubator in the intensive care unit. Throughout childhood, he suffered from physical illnesses; a pituitary deficiency was treated over many years with growth hormones; his scoliosis entailed long periods in hospital, and he was an in-patient for a year between 12½ and 13½ when he had the surgery. All his developmental milestones were delayed: walking at 19 months, talking at 2½, soiling until 5 or 6, and occasional bed wetting until age 9–10 when he finally achieved being dry at night. He attended a normal primary school, transferring to a special school for children with learning difficulties at 11. This was both to provide for his learning difficulties and to give him a more sheltered experience as his physical conditions made it impossible for him to survive the rough and tumble of a mainstream secondary school. He left school at 18 and completed a special foundation course for young people with learning difficulties at college. He did not want to return there and, at referral, was at home, unemployed.

Stanley's mother, in her late 40s, worked for the local authority. She had been depressed at his birth, worried about his physical health and survival, and in a marriage that did not survive beyond Stanley's third birthday. His father, an ex-soldier, had since the divorce worked at several jobs with no great tenacity and often borrowed large sums of (unrepaid) money from his ex-wife. Stanley could see him 'When I want to' but had not done so for over a year. The possibility of identifying with a weak and uninterested father might, therefore, be problematic.

Jim's arrival caused major change. A divorced former policeman, once very active on the folk-singing scene, he entranced Stanley with his tales of and friendships with well-known entertainers. At times Stanley could not help but enjoy this contact with the famous; at others, he remembered to dislike Jim as he had altered the mother–child dyad irremediably. Jim was concerned about Stanley's social isolation and successfully encouraged his involvement in a local drama group, performing and writing.

Thoughts on theory

In 'Three essays on the theory of sexuality' (1905), Freud outlined his view of fetishism:

> What is substituted for the sexual object is some part of the body (such as the foot or hair) which is generally very inappropriate for sexual purposes, or some inanimate object which bears an assignable relation to the person whom it replaces and preferably to that person's sexuality..........
> The situation only becomes pathological when the longing for the fetish passes beyond the point of being merely a necessary condition attached

to the sexual object and actually *takes the place of* the normal aim, and, further, when the fetish becomes detached from a particular individual and becomes the *sole* sexual object. (Freud S, 1905:pp.153–154)

The process of repression and idealization, and the splitting of the ego in the service of the defence against castration anxiety are fully elaborated in 1915, 1919, 1927, 1940/38a and 1940/38b.

Campbell (1989) describes work with 'Charles', an adolescent who first came for help at 16 and who finally sustained three years of five-times-weekly work from age 19. He outlines a history of abandonment and intrusion by the mother, an absent father, the development of a fetish for big-breasted (phallic) women as a defence against castration anxieties and suicidal wishes consequent on the sense of abandonment. Charles's phallic-oedipal conflicts centred around rage with the father for leaving him with his mother, and anxious competition with this father. The combination of early anxieties (abandonment, merging), castration anxiety and phallic aggression appear as key features.

Other descriptions of fetishism in children (Sperling, 1963; Wulff, 1946) seem more of transitional objects (Winnicott, 1951) and not fetishistic objects. Where a sexualized or displaced erotic relationship (e.g. with the mother's feet or shoes) is actually involved, there appear to be very few case examples of children in print. Sperling states:

> It seems to me that the need for a fetish has something to do with the reality of the child's experiences. ... there has been real seduction and actual over-stimulation of these component instincts in the relationship with the parents, especially with the mother. (Sperling, 1963:p.381)

This comes close to the role of trauma, perceived by Khan (1979) in the formation of perversions and by Hopkins (1984) in the formation of a foot and shoe fetish in her young patient with gender dysphoria. To Khan, the intrusion of the environment is a reality in the histories of many perverse patients, rather than the fantasy expressed by most neurotic ones, and this has often been a sexualized and sexualizing environment. Hopkins' little girl had been abused by her father.

Gaddini, developing Winnicott's work on transitional objects through her exploration of their precursors, has interesting comments on the infantile fetish, a pre-object stage phenomenon:

> 'The infantile fetish may be the temporary filling of a void caused by sudden loss.
> ... to do with the object and specifically the nipple. ... The infantile fetish
> represents a part object and not a function in relation to a person'.

And: '... castration (in terms of anxiety about self-loss) is basic to the structure of the infantile fetish'. (Gaddini, 1985/2003:p.57)

I find this useful, that castration is equated with overwhelming anxiety about loss of self which must be defended against. We find similar thinking in Ryan (2005).

Issues of separation and aggression also feature in the writing on fetishism. Siskind (1994) presents work with a 3½ year old who will not give up his nappies. Although resistance to nappy removal is not a prelude to fetishism, there are valuable comments here. Becoming a separate, autonomous person and gaining a safe capacity to use the aggressive drive were key themes in the work with child and parents. Aggression also features in Gillespie (1940, 1964), Coopersmith (1981) (who describes aggression subsequent to separation) Anna Freud (1965, 1966, 1972), Parens (1989) and in Campbell (1989), and difficulties with phallic aggression and potency. The need to keep the powerful maternal object at bay is also a theme, by dehumanization (Cooper, 1991), as a defence against aggression or against merging and being engulfed (Rabain, 2001; Ryan, 2005). Managing the transition of separation is key to Rabain's paper.

The role of the absent or passive father in the establishment of perversions has been noted by several commentators (Mancia, 1993; McDougall, 1995). Finally, Glover (1933) first drew our attention to the link between perversion and the development of the reality sense and so to perversion as a defence against psychosis. Coltart's case study also explores such a defence (Coltart, 1967/1996). I have found this to be the case with several adolescent gender dysphoric patients (Horne, 1999). It is noticeable that, in a somewhat polymorphous presentation, Stanley also cross-dressed at one time but that this appears not to have contained his anxieties.

When we think about Stanley's history, we see a child for whom the development of a sense of muscularity and body-self, the precursor in Winnicottian (1950–55) terms to positive aggressive affect, was grossly constrained. Indeed, his functioning at present indicates great inhibition in aggression. Separation was both enforced in an untimely manner (by hospitalizations and his mother's depression) and paradoxically also impossible to achieve. From the age of 3 he had no functioning oedipal third who might protect against merging or offer opportunities for identification, directing the child to the external world, away from the over-closeness of the mother–infant dyad. This continued in adolescence when issues of intimacy and sexuality must have required Stanley to seek a safe position away from this revival of closeness, when the potency of adolescent sexuality became an issue. The absence of a father, or adult sexual partner of his mother, appears to have left him with only the desperate manoeuvre of adopting a perverse solution. To keep the phallus safe, it became hidden in the merged pregnant mother dyad; to exercise his aggression and rage, he triumphed over the object by becoming it; in order not to deal with separation and mourning, he denies the need of an object. Work was patently not going to be easy, nor would it be swift.

Themes from the therapy: progress and process

Stanley is a short, slightly bent young man with brown hair that often sticks up in an unattended kind of way. He has poor articulation in his arms and finds shaving and combing his hair difficult. He dresses quietly but appropriately and can have a very lively look in his brown eyes. When he moves, he does so at speed. The large backpack that he brings (containing many drawings and folders of his main and symptomatic preoccupations) adds to a crustacean-like look.

He had three individual assessment sessions; I met his mother and Jim two weeks later, then had a final meeting with Stanley to discuss our way forward. He seemed spontaneous and quite definite about coming for therapy but when I asked gently what he would hope for from it, he could not answer. He pointed silently to his portfolio of pictures. I wondered aloud if there was, in the preoccupation with mummies and babies in his drawings, something about himself – who am I and what happened when I was growing bigger? He looked but could not answer. I also wondered to myself if there was, in his choice of therapy, less a collusion with his mother and Jim, or a wish for change, but more an aggressive attack – see, I have a therapy mother now and do not need to think about you. I noted that he always said 'mother' in rather a cold fashion. This could mean that the fact of having therapy might become important, rather than any change it might bring. Thus as 'subjective object' (Winnicott, 1962) I might further become a fetishistic object (Renik, 1992).

Brought by his mother or Jim initially, after eight weeks Stanley began to travel to therapy on his own (quite a distance from outside London by bus, train and underground) and has done so ever since. The work has been slow. Early themes were of being both mother and infant – a pregnant mother – with no need for an object and, crucially, no need to be angry or to mourn separation. He brought sheaves of drawings of pregnant mothers and a recurring dream of being a pregnant woman. Although he occasionally brings dreams, Stanley is unable to associate to these, stating them almost as concrete facts. His many drawings can go through several incarnations: he keeps his 'originals' and often copies them, then sees how they can be developed. I have taken up this idea of how things were in the beginning (his 'originals') and what can creatively be made of them.

A little history emerged from time to time but mainly he was in the here-and-now – or in the fantasy of his drawings, which to him appeared to have a reality. He had NO recollection (he was very firm in this, so firm as to be totally unbelievable) of his times in hospital. Eventually he was able to tell me a little of his school experience where there had been a good male teacher whom he could appreciate and whom he felt liked him too, but also, swiftly, a recounting of a bad male teacher, as if the first were too much to hope for. It had been hard to contemplate male identifications. Later, he did say that he had been unwell from time to time throughout school and I could connect it both to his spells in hospital and to a worry, perhaps, that therapy might make him unwell, challenge the homeostasis of his defences. He added that he has asthma and tires easily. In the transference, I took this as a warning about pace and survival.

The pictures of mothers and babies continued to appear, brought in large folders in his heavy backpack. The mothers, initially, were well-known female personalities whose glossy sexuality was important in their presentation and I wondered about the interest in 'infantile-mothering' concealing interest that was 'adult-sexual', almost like a sleight-of-hand deception: 'I have actually drawn this (a sexual picture) but I make you focus on that (a mother and baby)'. Soon a new drawing appeared, Tanya and her son Luke, Stanley's own invention, whose story centred mainly on their feeding and nappy-changing relationship. Tanya had blond hair, long red fingernails and a tendency in his drawings to look outwards 'to camera', even when ministering to Luke – a narcissistic mother, her nails potentially predatory. There was a striking lack of fathers. Then Tanya's home appeared – almost a mediaeval castle, impregnable and guarded by one armour-clad soldier outside a solid door. I asked, rather mischievously, if this were Luke's father, but no. There was no external third, protecting the male infant from being merged or damaged. After some months, we moved to whether Tanya wanted the infant for himself, as a separate person in whose individual capacities she took delight, or whether he was somehow an extension of her, the only man she needed, and thus not really a little boy in his own right.

In relation to this theme, I have found myself drawing greatly on my experience of parent–infant observation, but also on the ego structuring, developmental work long undertaken at the Anna Freud Centre, London, and described by Hurry (1998). This entailed asking what each was thinking of the other, what was in Luke's mind when he smiled or seemed apprehensive (as he increasingly did at nappy changing time), how he knew his mother was thinking about him – as if we were jointly the observers of the developing Luke. Stanley watched a television series on child development and read old books on infancy that he found in charity shops. He began to include aspects of attunement, gaze, Tanya reassuring Luke with her voice, as the central importance of Luke as a person was slowly allowed to appear. It felt as if there were times when a boy baby could begin to be safe and even enjoyed.

Some sixteen months ago – in the second month of treatment – Stanley let me see a page printed from the internet. It was for the 'Hubbies' web site, for hubbies (husbands) and naughty babies – patently a site for adult nappy wearers and also having something of the dominatrix about it – phallic women and men as babies. I offered rather obviously that this print out was very different from the adverts for Pampers and Milton that he had often brought or drawn. He nodded. I said that he found this exciting and he agreed. Stanley said he has a 'Big Babies' Kit' that he sometimes wears in bed at night under his pyjamas. I wondered about the sensations this gave – 'I don't really know'. I was thinking of skin and the kind of memories his traumatized body might have, plus the hidden sexual excitement in the nappy. 'I don't really know' means 'I am not yet ready to think about this'. He did, however, accept a comment about the importance of grown up baby men and strong women in his mind.

The drawings of a pregnant Tanya became less about Tanya and more about Luke – a large arrow labelled 'ME' pointed to the inside of the womb when she was drawn pregnant. I began to feel we were skirting around what had gone wrong, via looking at what was necessary for things to go right for the baby and, by displacement, Stanley. Luke's toys came alive when Tanya and Luke were not there – a sense that Stanley could be potent and mischievous when on his own.

Ambivalence towards Jim emerged at times. There was the beginning of enjoyment of conversations with him, and an appreciation of things Jim does for him. 'I don't really like Jim' came almost in the same breath and Stanley was able to talk about the disruption to him, alone with mother, when Jim arrived – but that some things about Jim were also very interesting. Developmentally, this certainly offered possibilities.

Stanley moved into the outside world eight months into therapy. He was offered a specialist placement at a Day Centre, a unit helping young adults with learning difficulties to prepare for work. He went there every weekday except his therapy day. There he aligned himself with the staff, finding the indiscipline of another group member very hard to take and reacting like a seven-year-old who struggles with superego issues: 'He did it and he shouldn't!'

His drawings began to contain little bug-like figures ('microbes') who were harmless to Luke and lived on the contents of the dirty nappies. His soiling until 5 and bedwetting until 9 or 10 meant his being in a nappy at night and must have given rise to a confusion of anal, phallic and sexual development. His anality is accessible in the microbes and additionally they perform the function he needs a non-narcissistic mother to perform – unlike the 'out to camera' mother of his first drawings, they can tolerate and appreciate his mess and the sense of agency and aggression that is bound up in anal interests.

After nine months of therapy, there was a brief glimpse of heterosexual masculinity in Stanley's choice of *Titanic* as his favourite film, although there followed a swift retreat into more childish choices. I was ill at the first session after Christmas: Stanley did not get the message and made the long journey to the clinic to find me absent. He could not access his anger or disappointment at this. Later that term, in March, I succumbed once more to 'flu. This time the message cancelling got through. Stanley came to the following session complaining of overwork and tiredness, and the demands of his week including his therapy. The Easter break loomed, as did Stanley's 21st birthday. He announced that he and his mother were having a holiday at his birthday (the last session before the Easter break) and he would not be attending.

On his return, he had drawn his usual pregnant mother but suddenly she was in a nurse's uniform – a nursery nurse, he said. I wondered if this was a screen memory of hospital when he was born, or an acknowledgement of his painful year there at 12/13. There was also great potential in straightforward male fantasy about nurses! She was, however, clearly wearing my shoes. I did not know how to take this up but there they were. I felt guilty I might be producing a foot fetish in Stanley... Part of me felt amused (the dangerous collusive reaction), part felt assaulted (he has stolen my shoes – he doesn't want my thoughts but will take over my shoes). I reflected on his need, faced with a longer break than expected, to retreat to female identification and part-objects. In thinking about this development, the desperation and aggression within it, and the beaming idealization Stanley shows when I come to collect him to start his session, I was greatly helped by Renik's article on the patient's use of the analyst as a fetish (Renik, 1992).

Some 14 months into therapy Stanley brought a dream of a woman with one breast covered and one exposed. There followed drawings over two sessions and, for the first time, he drew in the session what he had dreamed. There is nothing infantile about his drawing of breasts and it was possible to interpret that the breasts were of importance both to babies and to young men of Stanley's age who would see them as very sexual. He nodded. I commented on how appropriate it was for, say, a 21-year-old Luke to find this a sexy and exciting drawing. He stared at it. He agreed it was exciting but covered it over with baby drawings. I thought that sometimes it felt safer to think of 'baby Luke' rather than 'young man Luke with exciting thoughts'. He began to put the papers away: it was, unfortunately the end of the session and I awaited the return of his sexy lady for several months.

During one session in which it became very evident that, when I had a failure of attunement and he felt angry, Stanley had to take refuge in a defensive fantasy of merging ('I dreamed of you last night!') or fetishism ('You wanted me to be a woman' – like you), he succeeded in responding energetically to my talking of his anger and his need to be heard. At the end of the session, leaving the room, still in the basement, he said, 'See you next week'. At the start of therapy he never said goodbye, and, indeed, did not say hello but arrived and began, as if to deny any breaks and abandonments. For the previous six months he had said, 'See you next week' upstairs as he exited the clinic, the words addressed straight ahead of him to the main door. Now we could be separate, be seen to be so, and still be safe.

The next week we were back to the backpack and the safety of many drawings. He told me carefully that most were done on the two days prior to his session and I wondered if this could be connected – he needed the drawings less after our meeting but, when he was thinking about coming, he found the urge to draw. He looked at me silently, his brow wrinkled in puzzlement. The drawings were of nappy changing. The far more in-tune mothering was still very evident and I was able to make two interpretations – one about what might be in Luke's mind as the red fingernails approached him: 'It's my penis, don't hurt it and don't steal it'. This resonated with him and got a lively nod and smile. The second was to connect his frustration of the previous week about his work experience setting and schedule and the adults not hearing or being in tune with what he had said he needed, unlike Tanya who now knew how to be in tune with Luke.

Issues in technique

Monitoring the countertransference, using colleagues for thought, avoiding counter-transference acting-out (Baker, 1994) – all have been important in work with Stanley. To this Chasseguet-Smirgel (1981, 1985) adds the difficulty in establishing a therapeutic alliance, and the avoidance of insight and of the achievement of reality. This I have found with Stanley as I suddenly experience anxiety about being treated as an idealized but part-object – e.g. in the emergence of my shoes in his drawings, I wondered if his control over my difference, our individuality and his aggression takes the form of incorporating me. The pressure is thus to collude with the deception. I find something similar happens when my mind drifts. Usually, when this occurs with other young people, I find I am actually thinking of something that illuminates the therapy. With Stanley, I drift, and my mind is unconnected to the material. Here, colleagues have been helpful in pointing out that it is the phallic self being hidden again, a process of blocking me out from seeing his potency, and I can now use this as a cue for thought. Interpretations are often met with blankness, 'I don't really know' and rarely the sense I have offered something of meaning. At a later date I might have one fed back to me, as we all experience from patients when an interpretation has been meaningful and assimilated. With Stanley, it is hard to know at times if this has real internal meaning or if it is a rather adhesive identification with me. As the ego structuring work (especially affect recognition and legitimization) continues, however, I think that there *is* a slow, gradual pace of genuine internalization.

Much of the work has been done in the displacement of Luke and Tanya – it has been important to work on some of the anxieties in this manageable arena, approaching the affect gradually, slowly bringing it into the real world and the transference. With such a concrete approach and such perilously sensitive anxiety about castration and potency, Stanley has needed great care about pace and timing.

Several commentators mention the pressure to collude, to be a voyeur (McDougall, 1978), with 'the focus on the activation or enactment of the underlying unconscious fantasies in the transference' (Kernberg, 1997:p.30). This is very hard in the countertransference and seems connected to my moments of absence and the pressure to ignore his age-appropriate phallic potency. Re-reading the session material, I can see how swiftly, when I am not in touch, he initiates the female or infantile defence, and how long it can take for me to feel back in a comprehending mode.

Carignan has written that the passivity of analytic neutrality can be misconstrued as 'a repetition of early parental permissiveness and tacit encouragement of perverse behaviour' (Carignan, 1999:p.911). Stanley's mother 'did not notice' Stanley's flight from genital sexuality – and may well have colluded with it – until the arrival of Jim whose concern (as a male) activated help. I find I constantly struggle as to how active to be – when to leave silences, when these become collusive with a fantasy of being merged, and when to intervene. There are times when, to Stanley, people are merely impingements – and often ego-threatening ones. The issue of how the ego protects itself from intrusion and abandonment at the same time is a crucial one in the therapy and one that also affects my thinking about silences.

In the first nine months of work, there were very few indications of anger and aggression; I would be greeted with a beaming smile. I wondered if we would ever be able to access aggression and a sense of agency. My illnesses by chance helped open up the possibility of anger and demonstrated the threat that this presented to the immature self. Stanley wished to stop but could not quite put it in such aggressive terms! He was tired with being at the Day Centre, signing on at the Job Centre every fortnight, and then coming here. It was all too much for him and – exhaustedly – was making him ill. I sympathized with this, and commented on the great number of women who made demands of him – the staff at the Day Centre, his mother who found the place there for him, his experience at an earlier placement in a residential home for the elderly, and, of course, me who seemed to take for granted his coming here but who had let him down very badly by being off ill. I interpreted his great disappointment in me and how hard it was to hope that he could express the rightness of his annoyance.

When one thinks of the fetish as a response to trauma (Khan, 1979; Hopkins, 1984) one recalls Stanley's early experience of traumatic birth, unavailable worried mother, his not being the son his parents must have anticipated, his painful months in hospital, especially those when he was entering puberty, abandonment by father, and failure to grow. He has had multiple traumas. Additionally, one wonders about the mother of any child who stays in nappies at night until the age of 9 or 10, and what the child might mean in his maleness that has to be so hidden. The role of mother as narcissistic predator appears in his drawings – the hands with long red varnished nails reaching anonymously into the cot where baby Luke looks growingly apprehensive. It is not surprising that allowing the memory of such a traumatic childhood into his mind is as yet barely possible for Stanley. As we develop a kind of treatment alliance, and if in the transference I can gain stability as a reliable, non-threatening, valuing object, we may be able to get to the traumas. For the moment, I carry them in my mind and merely elucidate manageable aspects of them.

Stanley had adopted a position of not needing people and of not mourning the developmental achievements of individuation and separation. He could not entertain a sense of 'going on being' (in himself or his object) but appeared to insist on existing in the moment, denying separation or our week apart between sessions. This precluded both development (necessitating the fetish as the only route for sexuality) and reflection (the idea of the 'third' so well outlined by Britton, 1989). I have had to think carefully about intimacy and distance, taking care to engage him in the waiting room, where I greet him; and in the therapy room, when he rushes for his papers as we sit down, I ask how he is. This makes him pause, reminding him of our separateness. Sometimes he brushes it aside as if unheard, but more often now he will respond in kind. At times, increasingly, he can manage not to reach for his drawings. I see this as progress – I hope it means that, although he anticipates a predatory narcissistic object, he can be brought back in touch with a potentially benign yet separate one. He can now spontaneously tell me of aspects of his week – we *have*, then been apart – and how he felt. Moreover, his 'sexy lady' has returned, allowing a sense of phallic potency into the therapy room, with an apparent diminution in castration anxiety. Two weeks ago, after a long gap, he brought a further drawing of Luke. He was grinning, crawling on the floor, and his mother was in an armchair, reading, at an appropriate distance from him. 'I thought I would draw it for old times' sake', said Stanley. We thought together about the boy child, growing up knowing it was all right to be a boy. Stanley smiled and put Luke away in his folder.

Conclusion

We have a long way to go: the work is slow, not easy, and relies greatly on monitoring the countertransference. Stanley, fortunately, seems glad to continue. His mother and Jim have noticed significant change – Stanley is now willing to engage with the external world (he has recently gone back to college) and is much more communicative at home. He and Jim have a good working relationship. Having a father who claims him as male matters – Stanley's ambivalence is receding. The 'real world' advent of a benign, interested man, directing Stanley's interests outward and away from the terrifying and seductive need for merging, has complemented therapy where there has been little mention of his drawings and his interests are more latency ones.

The fetishistic position for Stanley, with its early, polymorphous presentation, has helped hold the abandoned fragile self with a solution that could contain the inexpressible rage with the object, conceal the growing sexual self, but which inhibited development and genuine potency. Thinking developmentally and analytically has been important and will be for some time to come.

Note

1 An earlier version of this paper appeared in the *Journal of Child Psychotherapy* (2003) 29.

References

Baker, R. (1994) Psychoanalysis as a lifeline: a clinical study of a transference perversion. *International Journal of Psycho-Analysis.* 75 (4), 743–753.

Britton, R. (1989) The missing link: parental sexuality in the Oedipus complex. In: Britton, R., Feldman, M. & O'Shaughnessy, E. (eds.) *The oedipus complex today: clinical implications.* London, Karnac.

Campbell, D. (1989) Charles: a fetishistic solution. In: Laufer, M. & Laufer, M. E. (eds.) *Developmental breakdown and psychoanalytic treatment in adolescence.* New Haven and London, Yale University Press.

Carignan, L. (1999) The secret: study of a perverse transference. *International Journal of Psychoanalysis.* 80, 909–928.

Chasseguet-Smirgel, J. (1981) Loss of reality in perversions – with special reference to Fetishism. *Journal of the American Psychoanalytic Association.* 29 (3), 511–534.

Chasseguet-Smirgel, J. (1985) Creativity *and perversion.* London, Free Association Books.

Coltart, N. (1967) The man with two mothers. In: *The baby and the bathwater.* London, Karnac Books 1996.

Cooper, A. M. (1991) The unconscious core of perversion. In: Fogel, G. & Myers, W. (eds.) *Perversions and near-perversions in clinical practice – new psychoanalytic perspectives.* New Haven & London, Yale University Press.

Coopersmith, S. E. (1981) Object-instinctual and developmental aspects of aggression. *Psychoanalytic Review.* 68 (3), 371–383.

Freud, A. (1965) Normality *and pathology in childhood: assessments of development.* New York, International Universities Press.

Freud, A. (1966) The *ego and the mechanisms of defence.* London, Hogarth Press.

Freud, A. (1972) Comments on aggression. *International Journal of Psycho-Analysis.* 53, 163–172. Reprinted in *Psychoanalytic Psychology of Normal Development.* London: Hogarth Press 1982.

Freud, S. (1905) Three essays on the theory of sexuality *SE* 7. London, Hogarth Press. pp. 123–245.

Freud, S. (1915) Repression. *SE* 14. London, Hogarth Press. pp. 141–158.

Freud, S. (1919) A child is being beaten – a contribution to the study of the origin of sexual perversions. *SE* 17. London, Hogarth Press, pp. 175–204.

Freud, S. (1927) Fetishism. *SE* 21. London, Hogarth Press. pp. 147–157.

Freud, S. (1940/1938a) An outline of psycho-analysis: Chapter VIII – the psychical apparatus and the external world. *SE* 23. London, Hogarth Press. pp. 195–204.

Freud, S. (1940/1938b) Splitting of the ego in the process of defence. *SE* 23. London, Hogarth Press. pp. 271–278.

Gaddini, R. (1985) The precursors of transitional objects and phenomena. *The Journal of the Squiggle Foundation*. 1, 49–57. Reprinted in *Psychoanalysis and History* 2003 5 (1), 53–61.

Gillespie, W. H. (1940) A contribution to the study of fetishism. *International Journal of Psycho-analysis*. 21, 401–415. Reprinted in Sinason, M.D.A. (ed.) (1995) *Life, sex and death – selected writings of William H Gillespie*. London, Routledge pp. 57–69.

Gillespie, W. H. (1964) The psychoanalytic theory of sexual deviation with special reference to fetishism. In: Rosen, I. (ed.) *The pathology and treatment of sexual deviation*. London, Oxford University Press. pp. 123–145.

Glover, E. (1933) The relation of perversion formation to the development of a reality Sense. *International Journal of Psycho-Analysis*. 14, 486–504.

Hopkins, J. (1984) The probable role of trauma in a case of foot and shoe fetishism: aspects of the psychotherapy of a six-year-old girl. *International Review of Psycho-Analysis*. 11 (1), 79–91.

Horne, A. (1999) Thinking about gender in theory and practice with children and Adolescents. *Journal of the British Association of Psychotherapists*. 37, 35–49.

Hurry, A. (1998) Psychoanalysis *and developmental therapy*. London, Karnac.

Kernberg, O. F. (1997) Perversion, perversity and normality: diagnostic and therapeutic considerations. *Psychoanalysis and Psychotherapy*. 14 (1), 19–40.

Khan, M. M. R. (1979) *Alienation in the perversions*. New York, International Universities Press.

McDougall, J. (1978) Plea *for a measure of abnormality*. New York, International Universities Press.

McDougall, J. (1995) The *many faces of eros*. London, Free Association Books.

Mancia, M. (1993) The absent father: his role in sexual deviations and in transference. *International Journal of Psycho-Analysis*. 74 (5), 941–950.

Parens, H. (1989) Towards a reformulation of the psychoanalytic theory of aggression. In: Greenspan, S. I. & Pollock, G. H. (eds.) *The course of life vol. 2: early childhood*. New York, International Universities Press.

Rabain, J.-F. (2001) Angoisse d'engloutissement et scenario fetichique. [The anxiety of being engulfed and the fetishistic scenario]. Revue *Francaise de Psychanalyse*. 65 (5), 1625–1639.

Renik, O. (1992) The use of the analyst as a fetish. *Psychoanalytic Quarterly*. 61 (4), 542–563.

Ryan, T. J. (2005) Clothes maketh the man: transvestism, masculinity and homosexuality. *British Journal of Psychotherapy*. 22 (1), 57–69.

Siskind, D. (1994) Max and his diaper: an example of the interplay of arrests in psychosexual development and the separation-individuation process. *Psychoanalytic Inquiry*. 14 (1), 58–82.

Sperling, M. (1963) Fetishism in children. *Psychoanalytic Quarterly*. 32 (3), 374–392.

Winnicott, D. W. (1950–55) Aggression in relation to emotional development. In: *Collected papers: through paediatrics to psychoanalysis*. London, Hogarth Press 1975.

Winnicott, D. W. (1951) Transitional objects and transitional phenomena. In: *Playing and reality*. New York, Basic Books 1971.

Winnicott, D. W. (1962) The aims of psycho-analytical treatment. In: *The maturational processes and the facilitating environment: studies in the theory of emotional development*. London, Hogarth Press 1965.

Wulff, M. (1946) Fetishism and object choice in early childhood. *Psychoanalytic Quarterly*. 15, 450–471.

Chapter 9

Self-harm and the harm of others in adolescents

Tim Baker

Introduction

A Portman colleague recently reported that a new patient in his therapy group referred to it as a 'survivors' group for people who had been sexually abused. He was swiftly corrected by a more experienced patient who reminded the newcomer that they were patients at the clinic because of the sexual offences they themselves had committed.

Maintaining a simultaneous sense of oneself as a victim and perpetrator is not a straightforward task for the patient or for the professionals working with them. In a young offenders institution to which I consult the staff habitually refer to the prisoners as 'the men'; however in a reflective practice session which followed the suicide of one of the inmates they strikingly started to refer to them as 'boys'. This shift in language illustrated the way in which the suicide appeared to have caused the staff to switch from thinking of these prisoners as perpetrators to thinking of them as victims.

In this chapter, I compare my work with an adolescent boy who repeatedly raped his sister (undeniably a perpetrator) and an adolescent girl who made a serious suicide attempt and who was seen as a vulnerable victim. The former is from the mainly male patient group of Portman adolescents who have carried out sexually harmful acts; the latter was a resident at an in-patient adolescent unit where the patient population is largely female, the majority of whom will have carried out acts of self-mutilation and made suicide attempts.

Neither patient has an obvious double identity as a perpetrator and victim: the girl from the adolescent unit did not commit a crime against anyone else, and the Portman boy was not himself the victim of a crime. However I think the comparison between them is helpful because of the way it brings to light the victim within the perpetrator and vice versa. It is Welldon's (1991) model of perversion which draws attention to the shared features of these two patient groups who might otherwise appear to have little in common. She suggests that whilst men 'use their penises to attack and show hatred towards symbolic sources of humiliation' (p.85), in female perversion the whole body is the instrument of sexualized aggression and that the 'crime' is committed against the perpetrator's own body. Welldon's (1988:p.21) reasoning for this is that, in contrast to men, 'women's bodies are completely taken over in the course of their inherent functioning by procreative drives'.

In psychoanalytic terms, the word 'perversion' is used descriptively to refer to erotic activity that does not have as its aim genital sexuality (Motz, 2008). As Glasser (1979) points out, the word remains helpful from this descriptive point of view despite the fact that in general usage it has unfortunate pejorative connotations. Stoller (1975:p.4) suggests that perversions are primarily motivated by hostility 'a state in which one wishes to harm an object' and contain 'a fantasy of revenge hidden in the actions that make up the perversion and serves to convert childhood trauma into adult triumph'.

Another Portman patient succinctly expressed what lay behind his perverse use of erotic activity when he became able to articulate a wish to have said to his father about his downloading of child pornography: 'look what's happening to your kid, Dad!' The adolescents I describe in this chapter are attempting to have an impact on their parental figures. They do this through the perverse harming of a person whom their parents hold dear: their child. In the situations, I describe this comes in the form of self-harm, harm to a sibling, and the extremely effective self-harm that is inherent in becoming a sex offender. This perverse form of relating allows an individual to express their intense hostility towards their object, whilst simultaneously preserving the object (Glasser, 1979). Physiologically and emotionally, these adolescents find themselves on the cusp of separation and independence. However, because of their early experiences and trauma, they are not equipped to take the frightening leap towards independence and so, one way or another must cling to their attachment figures, for whom they may also feel intense hostility. A key element here is the way in which risk taking (an ordinary feature of adolescent development) is, as Stoller (1975) describes, also central to perversion because of the need to create excitement. I will explore how such perverse risk taking thus allows these adolescents to satisfy the development push to feel separate from their parents or parental figures whilst paradoxically keeping both parties ever more enmeshed.

Pietr and Zoe

I will use two clinical examples, Pietr and Zoe, as illustrations. However, for reasons of confidentiality, these figures are drawn from aspects of a number of different patients at the Portman Clinic and adolescent unit respectively.

Pietr

Pietr was referred to the clinic following his conviction for the repeated rape of his 13-year-old half-sister. Pietr was 15 at the time and did not receive a custodial sentence. There were two younger half-sisters (aged 11 and 9) and there was no suggestion that he had attacked them. Pietr never knew his biological father, and was brought up by his stepfather. However, it was not until he was 12 that Pietr learned that his stepfather was not his biological father. At the time of his psychotherapy, Pietr had been placed with a foster family.

Pietr's narrative of his early life evoked the stark cruelties of the world of fairy tales and their wicked step parents. He felt that he was treated differently to his half-sisters recalling instances in which he was punished by having to remain at home whilst the others went on outings, or by not being allowed to eat his meals with the rest of the family. On another occasion he recalled his half-sisters being taken to Poland to visit his stepfather's family whilst he remained at home. He recalled with bitterness being supervised to do his homework by his mother whilst his siblings played happily in the other room. Indeed a great emphasis was placed on education by Pietr's mother, and, even as an older child at secondary school, she would sit with him at his desk as he completed his homework.

There was something soft and gentle about Pietr's mannerisms and he was always courteous and polite. Although his appearance changed over the course of his therapy to that of a more ordinary teenage boy, he was at first, unfailingly smart and tidy. In describing his offence, Pietr awkwardly told me that he had been curious to know what 'it' (sex) would feel like. He had crept into his sister, Agnieszka's room and she had remained, frozen, apparently pretending to be asleep whilst, silently, he at first touched, and then went on to penetrate her. This continued intermittently in the middle of the night for over a year. It remained unclear as to what, had finally, caused Agnieszka to disclose what had been happening.

Pietr's psychotherapy was, in its early stages, characterized by material in which he was a victim of a situation in which he felt he had been misunderstood and unappreciated. There was something suffocating and interminable about the way in which these complaints were quietly delivered, and the way in which just as they would have seemed to have come to a natural end, they would then start again.

Zoe

Zoe, an only child, belonged to the class of patient described by Anderson (1997:p.75) where the 'seriousness of their disturbance' is not communicated prior to the suicide attempt. She had quietly sailed through her childhood picking up scholarships and awards. She was often described as 'sweet' by members of the nursing team at the adolescent unit who liked her gentle demeanour and sympathized with her intense awkwardness. She was on the fringes of the peer group at the unit, and was preoccupied with anxieties about being a 'boring' person.

It emerged that Zoe's mother had suffered a late miscarriage (at 21 weeks) prior to Zoe's birth, and it became clear that this constituted an unprocessed trauma for her. It also seemed likely that this was linked to the post-natal depression she suffered in Zoe's first year of life, and subsequent bouts of depression she had suffered throughout Zoe's childhood. Zoe's mother would often complain about Zoe's apparently constitutional quietness, and it became clear that she had an idea of a 'fun' mother–daughter relationship that simply was not possible with Zoe.

Zoe's suicide attempt, a major drug overdose, took place at the seaside town where her family owned a holiday home. Zoe described to me how, having taken the tablets, she had laid down on a deserted stretch of beach on a summer's evening, listening to music on her phone. Before she closed her eyes she sent a WhatsApp message to her best friend, telling her how sorry she was, and how much she loved her. She did not give her the details of her location, other than she was at the seaside, and it was a matter of Russian roulette (Asch, 1980), Campbell and Hale (2017) that this message was enough for emergency services to find her. Later, in her psychotherapy Zoe told me how she had been planning the suicide meticulously for some time, but had changed the weekend for which it was planned because she did not want her death to spoil the opening of the school play in which her best friend had a starring role.

As the psychotherapy progressed, it emerged that in the weeks leading up to the suicide attempt, Zoe had been having difficulties with her peer group. She had been particularly distressed by their cruel WhatsApp group conversations in which she received messages as a member of this group which referred to social events from which she was being actively excluded. In one session, Zoe began to tell me about an idea that she had held about 'coming back' as part of nature, as a seagull who lived forever flying high above the world. It turned out that this is what she had believed would happen, that she would merge with nature, when she took the overdose and laid herself out on the beach. Having told me about this, Zoe abruptly left the session.

In the following session, Zoe told me that she did not wish to come for any further psychotherapy as she felt my time could be better spent seeing somebody who needed my help more than she did, and who would be more 'interesting' for me anyway. Over the course of subsequent sessions, we came to understand that Zoe had been angry with my response to the revelation of her suicide fantasy. Although I had not had a chance to respond to her before she abruptly left the session, Zoe was able to articulate that she had thought that the expression on my face was dismissive of what she had been describing. She had felt humiliated.

Aggression

It did not feel quite real that either the slight and unassuming Pietr could be a rapist or that the quietly spoken, baby faced Zoe could inflict such sadistic cutting on her body that plastic surgery needed to be considered. In both cases it was hard on meeting them to connect their appearances with what they had done. This disjunction between their presentations and the concealed violence of their activities was encapsulated in the details of Pietr's offence and Zoe's attempted suicide.

Pietr vividly conveyed the essentially gentle, careful way in which he carried out the attacks. They came across as denuded of explicit violence and aggression. Both parties also reported that there was no attempt by Agnieszka to defend herself or stop the rapes from happening until she finally reported them. This seemed hard to understand, particularly given that there was no suggestion from either's account that she was frightened of Pietr or physically intimidated by him in their daily life. Perhaps, though, it is more straightforward to respond to an attack if it is explicit that an attack is actually being made. In other words, it is may be simpler to defend oneself against an act of explicit physical aggression than it is to defend oneself from acts of physical aggression that come masked in gentle, possibly loving and possibly pleasurable, caresses.

Zoe's suicide attempt can also be seen as a violent, hostile act which falsely portrays itself as loving and considerate. It can be understood as a 'revenge fantasy', in which a surviving self (the seagull) looks down with a sense of everlasting triumph over those friends who have excluded and wronged her (Campbell & Hale, 2017). In such a fantasy, Zoe attacks and triumphs over those friends by taking the role of the victim, and imagining them feeling guilty for what they have done to her. It is a fantasy that is wrapped in an almost exquisite passive aggression. In changing the date of the suicide so as not to spoil her friend's opening night, her message seemed to be: 'I am so unimportant that I will even delay the date of my suicide so that it does not clash with the date on which my much more popular friend will be loved and admired and applauded by others'. The finishing touch to the way in which this murderousness was wrapped in love and concern was the suicide message to the best friend in which she told her that she loved her. Perhaps too it was no accident that she used WhatsApp (the weapon through which she herself had felt attacked) to do this.

Both the suicide attempt and the rape, then, were acts of intense hostility towards others which purported to be loving and gentle, and which appeared to be personified in the presentations of Pietr and Zoe themselves. They also had a particular impact on their victims who were unable to deploy ordinary aggression to protect themselves. In the case of Zoe's friends, they would not have known that they had been attacked until after the event (the attempted or completed suicide); and even then how could how could they express their anger with her for, in effect, implicating them with murder when all she was doing was expressing her love and consideration of them. Similarly, Agnieszka only responded to the attacks on her after they had taken place. It appears possible that there was a sense in which she too did not realize that she had been attacked until after the event.

Aggression and the countertransference

Being on the receiving end of this type of velvet gloved aggression is a familiar experience at the adolescent unit. For example, in a reflective practice session with the teaching staff at the unit, a teacher described a recent scene in the reception area. One or two visitors to the unit were present, whilst the teacher was re-arranging one of the display cases. In the corner on a sofa was a patient complaining to her mother about various members of the nursing team. The teacher was outraged by these complaints which she felt were inaccurate. In the reflective practice session she spoke about the way she had felt unable to intervene. This seemed to be partly a matter of design: to do so would be 'rude', to admit that she had been listening to a 'private' conversation even if this conversation was in fact a very public conversation that appeared to be intended to be overheard. The teacher, a highly capable and normally assertive individual, described how she had 'taken' herself away from the situation as she felt so filled up with rage that she did not trust herself not to lose her temper or act 'unprofessionally'.

This scenario is typical of what I am trying to describe at the unit because of the way in which the patient's aggression is expressed through victimhood and complaint and in such a way that it forecloses any straightforward response. The completed suicide is the ultimate expression of this scenario, an act of passive aggression to which any response or retaliation is foreclosed and redundant. The teacher's vivid description of her counter-transference is also instructive. She describes a situation in which she feels filled up with rage but without any means of expressing it. This can be understood as a projection of the mental state of these young people: overwhelmed with aggression but terrified of the apparently devastating consequences of expressing this aggression.

This situation was echoed in the early days of Pietr's therapy which were characterized by his sense of victimhood and complaint, and by my countertransference response of dulled aggression: like the teacher I often found myself filled up with an anger which I longed to discharge whilst also feeling it would be dangerous to do so. Pietr's complaints were accompanied by a piety which mirrored Zoe's saintly depiction of herself. He would speak about his altruism before complaining (at some length) about the self-centred attitude of others. I sometimes found myself, in response, nursing an impulse to blurt out: 'But YOU raped your sister!' (Indeed, it was important also to notice and avoid the temptation to wrap up such an impulse to crush Pietr in an apparently helpful interpretation about his projected aggression that would have said the same thing, albeit in a gentler manner). There was, then, a sense in which I was being invited to crush Pietr by simply reminding him of what had brought him to psychotherapy in the first place. The invitation appeared to be to victimize him with the truth: this would then have meant that instead of being in touch with being a perpetrator he could settle again into the familiar emotional state of misunderstood victim. Thus, he seemed to try to provoke a paralysing impasse in which it was difficult to find a benign way to talk about the rape: there seemed instead to be a choice between placating him by not mentioning his rape of his sister or devastating him in a cruel and punitive way by doing so. A further factor here was the veiled threat of self-harm or suicide (a threat which was very present in the early days of his therapy) and the sense that if I dared to talk about the truth he might harm or kill himself.

In this sense the dynamics of my relationship with Pietr further mirrored the dynamics of the weaponizing of victimhood and complaint by the patient group at the adolescent unit, an arena often characterized by excessive grievance and where the mere mention of conflict or difficulty can often lead to complaints about being 'triggered' and with it the veiled threat of suicide and self-harm. Just as I experienced with Pietr, staff can feel paralysed by the threat of being the cause of such catastrophic damage. It is perhaps important to point out there that there is a delicate line to be drawn between the needs of these patients to feel that their rightful sense of injustice and victimhood has been heard, and the point at which this tips over into weaponized victimhood. As Anne Horne (20?) points out, it can difficult to address the perpetrator side of a patient's personality until their status as a victim has been recognized.

It is not the purpose the of this paper to describe the process of the psychotherapy itself, but it is perhaps worth mentioning that in working with Pietr, I found it helpful to put to him the dilemma that he seemed to repeatedly leave me with: that in presenting himself only as a victim, he avoided thinking about himself as an abuser and that in doing this he seemed to be inviting me to become his 'abuser' who would crush him by reminding him that he had also been an abuser himself; and that being crushed in such a way would allow him to return to his sense of being a victim. In a related way in working with Zoe, it became possible, and I think helpful, to reflect with her about the way she had attempted to express her hostility towards me by trying to kill off our relationship and suggesting it would allow me the time to see somebody more 'interesting'. It was possible to link this expression of hostility through the assumption of victimhood and altruism to the dynamics of her original suicidal act.

Acting upon the parent

The situation I have been describing, is one in which straightforward, protective aggression is somehow unavailable. The teacher in reception and Pietr's sister, both apparently assertive individuals in their daily lives, were unable to protect themselves. These patients seem to communicate and project an anxiety about the potentially catastrophic consequences of aggression, a notion almost of being endowed with special powers, as if one false move could lead to destruction. In a sense this was actualized in the situation Pietr created with his sister: finally, she pressed the button and blew up his life. This is linked to the early therapeutic situation with Pietr in which these kind of anxieties meant that, like the staff at the unit, I felt tightly controlled in terms of what I could say to him. This has echoes of Joesph's (1988) concept of 'near death' – a sense of something (the therapy) being kept alive but with no hope of any real development.

This constellation of ideas is illuminated and explained by Glasser's (1979) theory of the core complex in which he links anxieties about the consequences of aggression to the failure to work through 'very early developmental stages' (p.280), noting also how the 'increase of sexual drives at puberty' (p.300) can bring these matters to a head. This early developmental stage is one in which 'closeness and intimacy' is experienced as 'annihilating' but 'separateness and independence' is experienced as 'desolate isolation' (p.280). To be close is to be suffocated, to be distant is to be abandoned. Glasser describes the circular nature of this predicament: the extreme sense of abandonment can provoke a desire to be close to the primary caretaker (usually the mother) which in turn provokes anxieties about being suffocated and annihilated and so on. According to Glasser, this situation mobilizes the child's survival instincts in attempts to save the self from the threats of smothering on the one hand, and abandonment to starve on the other. However, the instinct towards ruthless self-preservative aggression against the mother is inadequate in the face of these threats because the child still needs the mother to survive. In other words, aggression which on the one hand is felt to be essential is also felt to be potentially catastrophic: the button must not be pressed.

The histories of Pietr and Zoe both suggest that they would have been likely to have struggled to work through these early core complex anxieties. Their relationships with their mothers could both be understood as being characterized by an intrusively attentive closeness in the sense that their mothers appeared to have a fixed idea of the way they wanted their children to be (Glasser, 1979). Pietr felt an enormous pressure to comply with his mother's unusually obsessive demands for academic success; he linked this to her acute awareness of her low social status and wish for him to match the achievements of her more successful friends. Zoe, on the other hand, seemed to feel under pressure to comply with her mother's conception of a fun, lively daughter. Clearly, this seems to have been related to the mother's loss of the baby prior to Zoe's birth, and her fantasies about this baby. As with Pietr, Zoe's seemed not to feel that she was seen, understood or valued for herself. In adolescence these anxieties began to be played out with her peers and Zoe's pathological jealousy of the lively, admired best friend, and her sense of being overlooked and abandoned by her peer group.

Both of these parents, then, appeared in their different ways to be overly and intrusively close to their children in the sense that they were involved in trying to make their children fit with a fixed conception of what they should be. However, this way of relating is also intrinsically under attentive, because – as was clear from the children's accounts – they did not feel seen, understood or valued for who they were by mothers who were absorbed in their own needs.

Pietr and Zoe are therefore unlikely to have been able to work through the anxieties related to closeness and intimacy because they appear to have been related to by their mothers as if they were parts of their mothers rather than as separate entities. This is inherently 'annihilating'. At the same time, their anxieties about independence and separation are likely to have been overwhelming and equally impossible to work through, because they seem to have experienced their mothers, at times, as intensely remote beings who could not see or remain in touch with their true selves in a meaningful way. This sense of being cast away and excluded is palpably enacted in Pietr's description of his exclusion from the rest of his family (at mealtimes or when they went on holiday to Poland) and in a different way by Zoe's chosen scene for her suicide, stretched out alone on the beach, like a castaway on a desert island, whilst in her fantasy her friend is at the centre of the warmth and applause of the opening night.

The way in which this situation, according to Glasser, might have mobilized an aggressive survival instinct is likely to have been compounded further by the sense of grievance Pietr and Zoe harboured towards their families. Pietr felt that his younger sisters were preferred to him. He felt a sense of injustice because of the way in which he would be the one to get into trouble over conflicts with his sisters, and for the way he would be punished by being excluded from the rest of the family. At the same time, it is clear that Zoe had a powerful sense that a less concrete, fantasy sibling was preferred to her. Furthermore, anxieties about the consequences of their grievance and aggression are likely also to have been further exacerbated by the way in which (as became clear in the work with them) Pietr and Zoe saw their maternal objects as fragile. Pietr also reported that he was frightened of his mother's temper. In other words, any straightforward expression of aggression in relation to these grievances are likely to have felt dangerous because of either the risk of retaliation by the mother or the perceived danger of destroying her.

For Glasser, the solution to this overall predicament is the conversion of the aggression into sadism, by sexualizing the aggression towards the mother. In the sadistic attack, 'the aim is to control the object by inflicting pain and suffering' (Campbell & Hale, 2017:p.32). The individual is able to discharge their aggression towards their object without eliminating the object upon whom they are dependent for their survival. This perverse, sadistic solution is discernible in the therapeutic situations I have been describing, but, above all, in the scenarios of Pietr's rapes of his sister and Zoe's attempted suicide.

Zoe's fantasy of fusing with the seagull on the one hand, and, on the other, of being abandoned on the beach seems to be a vivid illustration of the core complex. Her suicide fantasy was not just, as I earlier suggested, a 'revenge fantasy', but also a 'merging fantasy' (Campbell & Hale, 2017) in which the patient believes she will fuse with an all-powerful mother nature. In this fantasy there is a splitting of the self from the body: the body is eliminated in order to allow this fusion. As Campbell and Hale (2017:p.48) suggest, this can be understood as a solution to intense core complex desires of fusion with the mother which bring with it concomitant anxieties about annihilation of the self: 'by projecting the hated engulfing, or abandoning primal mother onto the body and then killing it, the surviving self was free to fuse with the split off idealised, desexualised, omnipotently gratifying mother … a permanent sense of peace'.

This attempted elimination of the body is linked with 'ruthless aggression' as opposed to 'sadistic aggression' (Campbell & Hale, 2017; Glasser, 1979). However, there was also a powerful sadistic element in this situation which can be observed in Zoe's fantasy of triumphing over the guilt-ridden friends. Further, these friends – in Zoe's fantasy absorbed in their own fun, and not finding her sufficiently interesting – seem to clearly stand for her mother. At the same time, I want to draw attention to the sadistic <u>excitement</u> contained in this scenario. Zoe's WhatsApp message alerted her friend (and by extension her parents) to her overdose and that she was on the beach. The message contained no further information than this, and she had, furthermore, disabled the GPS function on her phone which would have allowed her to be tracked. She thus provoked a macabre game of hide and seek, in which the emergency services needed to race to find her before it was too late. I think that there was a perverse excitement in the idea of this 'game' (games are, after all, in their ordinary state designed to be enjoyed), and that in this it is possible to perceive the sexualization of the hostility towards the parent. As Campbell and Hale (2017) suggest of the psychological mechanisms that underpin self-mutilation, Zoe was using the threat to her body as an instrument of torture directed against the minds of her friends and parents.

A similar constellation is evident in the case of Pietr, although, of course the element of sexualization is displayed more prominently. The rape of his sister, then, can be seen as a sexualization of the profound hostility he felt towards his mother, a way of discharging aggression whilst preserving the object. There is a parallel with paedophilia here in which the inherently hostile, and spoiling attack that constitutes child abuse is clothed in the paedophile's often genuinely believed protestations of their love and reverence for children. The sexualized attacks are a way of expressing aggression and hostility without necessarily having to know (because of the dangers previously outlined) that this is what you are doing. Over the course of his therapy, and, in particular, in exploring his sense of exclusion in his new peer relationships, and linking the way these played out to the dynamics in his family, Pietr began to articulate his profound sense of grievance towards his mother. This hostility could then be linked to the rapes themselves.

The dynamics of the core complex can also be observed in Pietr's rape of his sister. The incestuous act itself might be understood as an expression of the desire for fusion with the mother (for whom the sister stands); the consequences of this act, once it was discovered, was a very real abandonment in that Pietr was removed from the family. One might speculate that these dynamics were played out in Pietr's mind over the year in which the rapes took place, with the anxieties about abandonment that he might have imagined he would suffer on discovery contributing to motivating the next rape and so forth. As with Zoe, harm (or the threat of harm) to the body of their child was used as an instrument of torture against the mind of the parent. Indeed to have their child rape a sibling would seem to be one of the most powerful, heart splitting tortures that any child could perpetrate against a parent. It is, furthermore, hard to think of what might constitute a crueller, more ruthless or apt revenge towards the parental wish to boast about the achievement of their children than this. In Pietr's case, then, there were two children being harmed. Primarily there was his sister against whom he used his 'penis[es] to attack and show hatred' (Welldon, 1999:p.21). However there was also a sense in which the aggressive impulse was turned inwards, and in Welldon's terms, in which he attacked his whole body. After all, there can be few more effective acts of self harm than causing oneself to be labelled a sex offender.

This overlap between these two distinct manifestations of perverse behaviour, which as Welldon asserts tend to be determined by gender, can be observed in other clinical examples at the Portman clinic and the adolescent unit. For instance, in thinking with another Portman patient about the way in which his downloading of child pornography might constitute an attack on his parents, he suddenly remembered that, at the time of this offence, he had also been drawn to downloading videos of 'real' deaths taken from headcams of people in accidents. We understood him, in viewing these images, to be in identification with these dying people and as having concomitant fantasies about the impact of this upon his parents. At the adolescent unit it is not uncommon to come across examples of teenage girls who will engage in a Russian roulette form of self-harm whereby they will meet, via the internet, in potentially dangerous locations unknown older men or women for sex. In a particularly apt variation of this, one girl was in the habit of meeting for sex, older women who physically repulsed her. It was a point of principle that these women would have an orgasm during these encounters, but that she would not. This, it seems to me, is a rather concrete illustration of a sexualized attack, and triumphing over, a symbolic parent. As with the viewing of illicit images on the internet, there is a key element here in the vital excitement derived here from the risk taking of meeting unknown older women via the internet. This excitement can be understood as part of the sexualization of hostility.

Hide and seek

It is joy to be hidden, disaster not be found. (Winnicott, 1963:p.186)

Winnicott (1963:p.179) comments that his concepts of being 'hidden' and 'found' could also be expressed in 'another language' as 'the fantasy of being eaten or swallowed up'. This, notably, brings us close to the language of Glasser and his ideas about core complex anxieties of being 'engulfed' by the object. Winnicott also discusses the way in which these issues are particularly urgent during adolescence since 'the individual... is not quite ready to become one of the adult community there is a strengthening of the defences against being found, that is to say being found before being there to be found' (p.190). Winnicott outlines the way in which the adolescent seeks to preserve a sense of himself or herself as an 'isolate' and how this is a necessary part of the search for identity. The paradox, as Winnicott so beautifully describes it, is that it is a disaster if having established such an identity it is not seen, known or indeed found by others.

Earlier, I suggested that Zoe's suicide message provoked a macabre game of hide and seek. Indeed it could be understood as a perversion of the childhood game and its joyous reunion, the: 'there you are!' of the delighted mother, and the squeal of 'here I am!' as the proud child reveals her body to her parent. Instead of producing a body to be admired, for Zoe there appeared to be a fantasy of producing a dead body with which to torture and shock her parents. Such hide and seek games are a familiar feature of the presentations at the adolescent unit.[1] A good example is another patient who used to hide in communal areas of the unit, literally 'playing dead' by lying completely still under a sheet or cushion. On one occasion when I came to get her for a psychotherapy session, it turned out that what had appeared to be a discarded shoe actually contained the foot of the patient.

Pietr's rape of his sister did not appear to carry with it the same invitation for his parents to 'seek' him. However, once the secret was discovered, the parents would have been confronted with a revelation concerning the bodies of their children which would have caused shock and torture rather than pride. Another Portman patient told me about his (unacted upon) sexual thoughts about his sister as he watched her sleep from her bedroom doorway and the sense of risky thrill attached to what he might do to her. He was able to articulate that the thrill was linked to the dangers of being caught. I think it is unlikely that such a risk taking excitement about the idea of being caught was not also present in Pietr's mind. In other Portman adolescent patients, furthermore, the invitation to be discovered is more readily observable – for instance, one boy who sexually exposed himself online was fully aware that his mother was anxiously monitoring his online usage. In these Portman examples there seems to be something shameful, and potentially repulsive, in how these adolescents' sexuality is 'found' by their parents. This is also familiar particularly in cases when adolescents have been found downloading child pornography. In these Portman cases, hostility towards the parental figures appears to be expressed through this aggressive, repulsing sexuality; this, I think is a counter-point to the use self-mutilation by the patients at the adolescent unit in which the body is revealed to the parental figure in a similarly repulsing and hostile way.

These presentations are, I think, a product of the conjunction of the adolescent process with its ordinary search for identity – to be both an 'isolate' and to be known – and the perverse sexualization of hostility towards parental figures that, as I have described, derives from unresolved core complex anxieties. This, in turn, is linked to the profound sense of not being valued for their true selves felt by both Pietr and Zoe, and their compliant 'false' selves. My experience of these patients is that, like Pietr and Zoe, they can often present with a sense of internal emptiness, an extreme version of Winnicotts 'being found before being there to be found'. This might be seen as an inevitable consequence of a parental failure of mentalization (Fonagy et al., 2003) and the parental inability to think about the mental states of these children, and so allow the children to know themselves for themselves. Therefore, it as is if there is a sense in which these patients define for themselves a true self that is in opposition to the false obedient, sweet, compliant self; in other words, in this vacuum the true self becomes (perhaps equally falsely) defined as intrinsically dark: repulsing, hostile and shameful. This I think links to the way in which self-mutilation can be motivated by an impulse to regain a feeling of 'being real' (Motz, 2008:p.218).

In describing their work with highly disturbed borderline adolescents at the Cassell Hospital, Flynn and Turner (2003:p.158) write that 'attainment of this sense of value is the single most important objective in adolescence'. This is both recognizable in the patient groups I am describing, and makes good sense. The adolescent needs to attain a sense of value in him or herself, including a sense of value in their new sexual body, in order to have the essential confidence to separate from their parents and manage adult life. In relation to this, it is perhaps worth pointing out that, in attachment terms, feeling not sufficiently interesting to a parent is likely to be experienced as a form of threat: after all if an infant does not capture the interest of a parent then there is the danger that the infant will not be protected by the parent – being 'interesting' in this sense is a matter of life and death. These perverse hide and seek games can thus also be understood as maladaptive responses to an attachment threat, containing an explicit, deadly challenge which goes beyond 'am I worth seeking?' into 'am I worth saving?' They express both hostility towards the object, and, at the same time, a need for the object's protection.

The different acts of Zoe and Pietr thus led to a situation in which they were both heavily monitored, and in which they were denied some of the ordinary adolescent steps towards independence. Pietr was placed on the sex offenders register, and he was regularly monitored by social care and probation. On some level, Pietr, like the other Portman patients to whom I referred above, could be said to have extended an invitation to parental figures to intrude into his sexuality; it is as if these patients are striking both forwards towards an independent sexuality and backwards towards a situation in which their bodies are under the jurisdiction of their parents. There is a concrete equivalent to this at the adolescent unit in the form of the intrusive observations, which sometimes include a lack of privacy in the bathroom and toilet, invited by the extreme suicidal risks posed by these (mainly) young women.

In a similar way both the rape and the overdose must have required a form of courage, a setting out on their own to do something new; in this respect they could be said to represent the adolescent pull towards independent functioning. In Zoe's case this newness was expressed in the notion of her 'ideas' about 'nature' – this came through in her sense of pride in having come up with these ideas, and the way she seemed to use them to express her individuality. Deadly as these theories may have been they still seem to contain a certain adolescent spirit of inventing something new, of breaking free from the established way of thinking. At the same time, repellent as Pietr's crime against his sister was, it, nonetheless, contained an element of genuine adolescent sexual curiosity, a wanting to know what it would feel like. Yet, as I have been describing, their actions led to Pietr and Zoe being supervised and monitored as if they were small children. Their actions thus meant they could delay the ordinary adolescent anxieties about surviving without such supervision, and could feel less pressure to develop independence. These actions therefore allowed them to discharge or express their developmental urges towards independence without having to suffer the anxieties inherent, for instance, in managing an actual sexual relationship.

In this respect, the activities of Pietr and Zoe provide a solution to their predicament in which they find themselves – compelled by their bodies and environments towards the adolescent task of separation and individuation, yet ill equipped to do so. Just as the sadistic solution to the core complex allows for the expression of aggression without eliminating the object, this way of operating allows for an outlet for the adolescent urge towards independence – in particular through risk taking and sexuality – without the need to endure the, as yet, unmanageable consequences of independence.

Note

1 In-patient units, and the way in which their residents are 'hidden away' from society is another determining factor here (Motz, 2008).

References

Anderson, R. (1997) Suicidal behaviour and its meaning in adolescence In: Dartington, A. & Anderson, R.(eds.) *Facing It out: clinical perspectives on adolescent disturbance. Tavistock clinic series.* London, Routledge.

Asch, S. S. (1980) Suicide and the hidden executioner. *International Review of Psycho-Analysis.* 7, 51–60.

Campbell, D. & Hale, R. (2017) *Working in the dark: understanding the pre-suicide state of mind.* London, Routledge.

Flynn, D. & Turner, J. (2003) In: Day, L. & Flynn, D. D. (eds.) *The containment of borderline adolescents in the internal and external worlds of children and adolescents collaborative therapeutic care.* Routledge.

Fonagy, P. et al. (2003) The developmental roots of borderline personality disorder in early attachment relationships: a theory and some evidence. *Psychoanalytic Inquiry.* 23 (3), 412–459.

Glasser, M. (1979) Some aspects of the role of aggression in the peversions. In: Rosen, I. (ed.) *Sexual deviation.* Oxford, Oxford University Press.

Horne, A. (2001) *Brief communications from the edge: psychotherapy with challenging adolescents.* Journal of Child Psychotherapy, 27 (1): 3–18.

Motz, M. (2008) *The psychology of female violence: crimes against the body.* Hove: Routledge.

Stoller, R. (1975) *Perversion.* New York, Pantheon.

Welldon, E. (1988) *Mother, Madonna, whore. The idealisation and denigration of motherhood.* London, Free Association Books.

Welldon, E. (1999) Psychology and psychopathology in women – a psychoanalytic perspective. *British Journal of Psychiatry.* 158, 85–92.

Winnicott, D. (1963) Communicating and not communicating leading to a study of certain opposites. In: The *maturational process and the facilitating environment: studies in the theory of emotional development.* London, Karnac 1965.

Chapter 10

'Securing the disaster zone. Assessing the damage. Sifting through the rubble'. The early stages of psychotherapy with a traumatized boy

Patricia Allan

> *Trauma victims cannot recover until they become familiar with and befriend the sensations in their bodies.*
>
> (Van der Kolk, 2014:p.100)

I recently watched a film that depicted a small town devastated by an earthquake. Most of the buildings had partially or fully collapsed. In one scene, scores of rescue operators were urgently trying to secure the remaining buildings so they could search for survivors. Looking at the carnage, it was hard to imagine they would find anyone alive in the rubble. Suddenly, someone called for silence. The dust-caked workers paused and switched off their machinery. There was an eerie silence......then a small cry for help......silence.....and then another cry which sounded as though it came from a child. Some of the workers rushed forwards in the direction of the child's voice. Others held them back, aware that before the child could be rescued, the remnants of the building had to be propped up and made safe, otherwise the rescue effort might cause further damage and endanger the child. The tension between the desperate urge to rescue the child and the need to pause, carefully assess the situation and plan how to do this safely, reminded me of the stages that a referral to the Portman clinic can go through, prior to the young person being treated.

When describing his work with juvenile delinquents Donald Winnicott (1964) spoke about how, when you encounter a disturbed young person, you are meeting a life that has gone wrong, usually very early on. Most of the young people referred to the Portman have lives that have gone wrong, usually very early on, and continue to do so. They have often exhausted other options – been to many schools, had multiple foster placements, different social workers and have been referred to a variety of mental health providers. The young people referred have entrenched difficulties, are emotionally bent out of shape and hard to be with.

The Portman clinic specializes in working with perpetrators. Referrals are often made in the aftermath of a disastrous enactment which has resulted in someone being harmed. The young person referred has 'breached the body boundary' and is now considered to be high risk. The network around them is tasked with managing the risk.

When we accept a new referral, our first step is to ensure that the young person is supported by a strong, effective network. This involves working with carers, educators, social services, youth offending services and other significant people in the young person's life. Just as the rescue workers in the film had to carefully calculate where reinforcements were required in order for the damaged building to be considered safe to enter, we work with networks to help them link together to comprehensively support their young person, thus making psychotherapy viable. If there is no existing network, we work to create one. There is often a hope that psychotherapy will help to manage the risk which the young person poses. This is not the case. If anything, starting therapy can de-stabilize the patient in the short term which is why it is vital that there is a cohesive network working together to understand the needs of the young person and create an environment which facilitates their social, educational and emotional development. It is only when we feel confident that this type of risk management is in place that we would arrange an assessment for psychotherapy.

Anna Freud helpfully said of her work with vulnerable young people

'first you have to build the house before you can throw anybody out of it' (Anna Freud, quoted in Sandler, Kennedy & Tyson 1980)

This idea, that some patients need the space and time to build a trusting experience with their therapist before their trauma can be addressed, seems particularly true of young people who are harmful to others. Anne Horne (2019), in relation to Anna Freud's metaphor, describes how ego development is the precursor to projective identification and how an emotion has to be discovered and named before it can be thought about and related to behaviour.

In my clinical work at the Portman, I have noticed a primal 'pre-building' therapeutic process which I have broken down into three stages. If we return to the image of the earthquake, the first stage would be to 'secure the disaster zone'. This begins with the referral and does not involve the young person but the professional network. The second stage I call 'assessing the damage'. This is an opportunity for the clinician to meet with the young person for a set number of sessions to begin to glean, through the young person's use of the setting and the clinician, their relational history and whether psychotherapy is a viable option. The third pre-building stage I call 'sifting through the rubble'. This is the process of gathering up the emotional debris of things which have gone wrong in the young person's life to date. As Anne Alvarez would say, we need to understand the 'what' before moving to the 'why' (Alvarez, 2012). If the 'what' involves pre-verbal trauma, the work may involve recognizing that bodily states are the patient's initial channel of communication. When this is the case, a physical rather than a verbal response is likely to be more containing for the patient. This may involve an adaptation of technique. Sifting through the rubble and finding a shared acknowledgement of these experiences means that they can be processed, thus clearing enough building space for new emotional foundations to be laid.

Referral

Sean, a young boy in foster care, was referred to the clinic by his social worker when he was eight years old. He had recently been excluded from school for sexually propositioning a female teacher, simulating sex whilst lying on top of a female classmate and hitting a male classmate over the head with a plank of wood when Sean was beaten by him in a game. Other disturbing behaviours at home included urinating and defecating in his bedroom, inserting his fingers and other objects into his anus, poking his eyes and nose until they bled, putting dangerous objects into his mouth, overeating, hoarding food and insomnia. His social worker was afraid that Sean was thought of in the network as a disruptive and aggressive child, rather than a traumatized child. The social worker was also afraid that the foster placement was being put under too much strain.

Sean came from an Irish Traveller background. At the time of his birth, Sean's mother was a class 'A' drugs user with mental and physical health issues. Sean was mother's sixth child. His father, absent since before the birth, died of a drugs overdose without ever meeting Sean. The moment Sean was born, he died and had to be resuscitated. He was addicted to drugs and had to go through withdrawal. Mother and Sean were then discharged to a mother and baby placement. Eventually, they were allowed to return to mother's home and were discharged from social services. Mother began to use drugs again. Sean grew up in a criminal environment where he was exposed to drug and alcohol abuse, violence, sexual violence and violent pornography. He was emotionally and physically neglected and abused and showed all the signs of having been sexually abused. He was trained to shoplift and to lie to anyone in a position of authority. After concerns were raised at school, he was taken into foster care aged seven. When we received the referral, he had been in his foster placement for 14 months. The foster carers were very committed to Sean and keen to understand his needs and support his well-being.

Securing the disaster zone

At the time of Sean's referral, the network around him was not joined up or robust enough to make therapy a safe option. Sean was out of school, his foster carers were not being given enough support in managing him and were losing confidence in their ability to do so. As Sean's isolation increased, his bizarre and destructive behaviours escalated.

The referral was initially taken by a colleague, Ms B, who brought the network together and worked with them to find a suitable school placement for Sean which had the resources to respond to his particular needs, both educationally and emotionally. Ms B also emphasized how important it was to provide more/better support for the foster carers. Gradually, each part of the network was strengthened and able to meet Sean's needs. With the right level of support, he was able to manage a new school placement. This gave the foster carers space and time to get on with organizing other aspects of Sean's life. He was supported in school to have appropriate contact with his peers and, as he began to feel more confident in the school setting, he was able to access learning.

Perhaps most importantly, Ms B was able to alter the network's perception of this child by helping them to link his early trauma with his current presentation. Whilst Sean had been referred to our service as a perpetrator it was important that the professionals acknowledge he was also a victim. This realization freed the network up to be curious about what Sean might be communicating through his disturbed behaviours and to think about what he was working hard to cover up in terms of loss. It took eight months before the network was able to provide the level of support needed for Sean to be accepted for an assessment for psychotherapy.

Assessing the damage

I first met Sean in a meeting with my colleague Ms B, his foster parents and social worker. He sat on a sofa tightly wedged between his foster parents, as though they were literally propping him up. He sat upright, shoulders up to his ears, hands interlaced on his lap, with a fixed smile. He spoke only to say words which did not seem to be his. For example, when asked what he thought about coming for therapy he said 'I think it would be good for me, a place to talk about my feelings' in a practiced tone. There was nothing spontaneous about him but a sense that he was holding everything in and working hard to present a 'good boy' version of himself. It was painful to witness. We agreed to begin an assessment.

Sean attended the assessment sessions as different characters. It felt as though I was meeting aspects of Sean's defences personified – the protectors of the helpless, frightened boy who was hiding under the rubble. He came to the first assessment session as 'good boy' Sean. Good Sean sat down in a chair and eagerly engaged. He was grateful and benign and saccharine. He enthusiastically agreed with everything I said and made no demands. I felt as though I was with a manic puppet, operated by someone outside the room. I felt wary and repulsed, but also worried that if Sean kept this up, he would fragment. I suggested he might want to play with some of the toys. He spent the rest of the session in silence, sitting on the floor with his back to me, making lego cars. As I watched him, I felt profoundly sad. At the end of the session, he handed me the two lego cars he'd made and, in a more authentic voice, asked if I would keep them for him until next time.

In assessment session two I was surprised to meet 'stupid' Sean. This Sean had a stumbling gait, held his arms and hands in front of him as though he was about to play the piano, and spoke with a sing-song tone, as though he had an enlarged tongue and a lisp. As he played with the lego he spoke to himself, describing what he was going to do and then what he was doing.

> *now, where does this one go? I'm so stupid.... Here? No, silly me, that doesn't fit. I wonder if there's another piece like this?........I can't find one, oh no, there is one......no, it's the wrong one...stupid*

This Sean filled the room with 'not being able to'. Any attempt on my part to engage with him evoked a glazed look and an apology that he didn't know what I meant because he was stupid. I experienced this as an act of powerful passive aggression. I felt frustrated and useless. At the end of the session, he handed me the two cars in silence.

Occasionally there would be a slip. During a 'stupid Sean' session:

> *Sean takes the lid off the play dough and tries to prise it out. He makes exaggerated grunting, huffing and puffing noises. He says "I'm going to make something now" in his sing-song, clumsy voice. He begins to describe a monster who has spikes on the outside and a scary face. I say that it would be hard to get close to someone like that – they might look as though they were tough, but they might feel lonely sometimes, and maybe they would like a better life. Sean is quiet and continues to shape the dough. I say that maybe Sean would like a better life and he nods. After three beats of silence, Sean straightens up in the chair, looks directly at me, squashes the monster into a ball and in his real voice says "I shouldn't have said that" as though I have tricked him.*

Sean was quiet for the rest of the session. As we were leaving the room, he let me know, in his real voice, that he didn't know what we were supposed to be doing but he felt today had been a waste of time. I felt as though I had made a clumsy attempt to prematurely look beneath the rubble. This resulted in Sean feeling emotionally intruded upon and exposed and left him feeling humiliated and ashamed. I became aware that I had to alter my technique in some way but was not sure how.

The most disturbing version of Sean I met was the 'perverse baby' Sean.

> *Sean sits on the floor at the side of my chair. He slumps to one side and leans against my left leg. I speak gently to him about how I think it is hard to be Sean sometimes. Maybe people see a boy who tries hard and who is quite tough, but I think sometimes they don't see how worried he is. I say*

that sometimes people cover up worried feelings by acting like a tough guy, but underneath the tough guy there might be a boy who wants to be able to relax and rest and not always be tough. I notice Sean's head is getting nearer to my groin and I feel uncomfortable. I ask if he would like to hear a story. He says yes. I pick up the cushion from the next chair and am about to put it between my groin and his head when Sean takes the cushion and says "this can be my teddy" and hugs it. He turns his head and smiles at me with a sexual invitation in his eyes. I feel shocked. I stand up and get the other cushion and use it for his head. It feels crucial that I put a barrier between his head and my groin.

The perverse baby was another of Sean's solutions in managing my attempts to look beneath the rubble prematurely, usually appearing when I said something that I hoped would be containing but which Sean experienced as intrusive and which provoked a defensive response. In this instance, Sean eroticized the aggression and invited me to join him in a perverse sexual coupling (Campbell, 2005). This way he could maintain the contact by controlling it. Again, I was aware that my attempts to put words to his experiences increased Sean's anxiety rather than alleviating it, but this time he had found a solution which was relational, albeit perverse.

Over the course of the assessment, I met many versions of Sean. There was no symbolic play-acting in his use of these constructed selves, nor did they seem to work together as a gang. It felt as though they were exaggerated, fragmented parts of him whose task was to keep me away from authentic Sean, the helpless victim. Each disguise showed me something about his internal world, his relationship with the external world and his need to be defensive. Gangster Sean would strut around the room and rubbish everything. Security Guard Sean would wear a paper mask sellotaped to his face, hold a weapon made from Lego and stand guarding the door, facing me, as though I was the person who must be kept out. Each version of Sean would speak to me and answer my questions, but our exchanges felt meaningless and his defences impenetrable. My attempts to acknowledge, understand and contain were experienced as hostile attacks. Sometimes the only straight forward exchange was when he silently placed the two lego cars into my hands at the end of each session. It was only in this wordless exchange that I knew that he wanted me to hold onto something for him and keep it safe.

Sean used language to hide from or avoid real contact and he mistrusted everything that I said to him. My counter transference suggested he was one of the most disturbed children I had treated. I also knew, absolutely, that he was desperate to have therapy, however mightily his conscious self might rail against it. We agreed to take Sean into treatment after the summer break. During the final assessment session, he insisted I make him an appointment card which he could take away with him, which showed the date and time of his next session. I felt rather pleased by this request and carefully made and gave him the card. It was quickly followed by:

Sean picks up a plastic bag and blows it up. He ties a knot and says "I'm going to leave you my breath". Taken by surprise, I look at him with a smile. He returns my look and holds my gaze as he, quite deliberately, bursts the bag of air. He looks down at the bag then back up at me saying, with a bambi-like innocence "uh-oh". I feel humiliated and stupid and thoroughly duped.

In terms of 'assessing the damage', Sean presented as a perverse, corrupted, violent and controlling little boy whose internal landscape was broken and scarred.

'Sifting through the rubble'

When working with Sean it quickly became apparent that words needed to be used carefully and that I was going to have to find a way to work with him that was not bound up in language. He was a very active patient and used his body as his main means of communication. My attempts to attach words to his actions usually failed. For example, he regularly built elaborate disaster zones in the therapy room and would then try to avoid annihilation by making risky moves from one piece of furniture to the next. When I tried to describe what I thought he was going through, Sean would stop. It felt as though my words pulled him back into a conscious defensive state which led to a shutting down. When I changed tack and added noises which I felt matched his actions, he silently acknowledged my contribution to his story and continued to act out his catastrophic experiences. The soundtrack of alarm and fear which I provided provoked a reaction which suggested he felt understood in a way that he did not when I used words. I realized that the process of sifting through the rubble would not be achieved by sitting and talking, but required sound and movement. Sean suffered trauma pre-verbally and I began to wonder whether there was a link between unprocessed pre-verbal trauma and the compulsion to use the body to communicate this experience physically rather than verbally. Certainly, when working with Sean words not only felt inadequate, they actually created a barrier to communication.

The experiences which Sean conveyed in the therapy room were vivid and, at times, almost unbearable. When confronted with the therapy box for the first time, Sean's reaction was to destroy it.

For the next 25 minutes or so he tries to break everything in his box. Cars are flattened, dolls dismembered and soft toys disemboweled. For most of it he wears an expression of a mad cartoon type character. The corners of his mouth are drawn back, revealing his teeth, his eyes are narrowed and his forehead furrowed. There are elements of a rabid dog, a smiling torture victim, a robot, but worst of all I see abject, humiliating terror which makes him look ancient. As Sean breaks things he laughs and congratulates himself. He ignores me, however if feels as though it is important to him that I am here to witness the extent of the damage he has experienced and can wreak.

This full-frontal attack on the box and its contents reminded me of the sustained attack Sean suffered in utero, as his Mother continued to abuse drugs throughout her pregnancy so that even the womb was experienced as catastrophic. As he moved from one abusive experience to the next, Sean seemed to have learned that his survival depended on sabotaging any possibility of meaningful contact or attachment, in order to control the inevitable ensuing loss (Morgan, 2007).

Sean was fond of using the soft ball to play catch with me; however, he found it difficult to sustain this joined up activity. He would complain that this 'calm stuff' was quite boring. After a minute or so he would think of something more difficult to do, for example, throwing the ball in the bin, thus moving away from a joint activity to a solo task. When he successfully got the ball in the bin, he would add another level of difficulty, putting the bin in a harder-to-reach place or throwing with his eyes closed. The task inevitably became impossible. I began to think that the 'calm stuff' – joined up, predictable and interactive – put Sean in touch with what had been unavailable from his Mother. Sean was then driven to re-enact his actual experience, a scenario where he fails to sustain a connection with a significant other. Sean and I shared moments of successful attachment, but they were quickly succeeded by an insurmountable barrier. Sean seemed stuck in a cycle of seeking perverse, exciting contact, all body and no mind, which was bound to end in failure.

When Sean failed in the game, he would hurt himself. Sometimes he would dive for the ball in a reckless manner guaranteed to result in injury. At other times he would bang his head against the wall or put something sharp in his mouth. When he thought I was annoyed with him he would hurt himself. When we faced a break from therapy, he would hurt himself. In the early days of therapy, I struggled to manage this self-harm. It felt manipulative and filled me with rage and helplessness.

Sean rummages through his box saying "where's the pen?". He finds the red felt tip pen and scribbles all over the face, hands and crown of the King puppet saying "there's blood everywhere, on the face, blood on the crown...." Sean keeps looking up at me, as though I am going to tell him off or stop him. He tries to scribble on the arm of the chair but the pen won't work. He looks at me as though I have won and throws the pen back into the box. He stands up and says "right, now I might as well kill myself" and comes over to my chair and tries to grab the blanket which is on the back of my chair. He can't dislodge it and lets it go. He grabs the lid of his box and begins to hit himself on the head with it, looking at me with fury and challenge. I say that he wants me to feel worried about him in case he really hurts himself. He whacks himself harder and I begin to feel mounting panic and a strong desire to look away.

The material above reminded me that Sean had died as soon as he was born and had to be shocked back into life. I wondered whether Sean felt compelled to re-enact his near-death experience (Joseph, 1982). As soon as he was brought back to life, baby Sean had to go through drug withdrawal. I used to work in a hospital and once observed a baby going through this process. The baby was inconsolable – continually crying jaggedly on the inhale rather than the exhale, as though even breathing was sore and the protest was directed inwards rather than out. Her limbs twitched and jerked uncontrollably. She continually punched herself in the face. Her back arched and fell, arched and fell. No one could stay with this baby for long. She was passed from one nurse to another but also spent a lot of time alone. Sean's behaviour when he thought something was wrong, had this disorganized self-attacking feeling to it. I found myself at a loss as to what to do. Scrabbling around in my mind for the perfect interpretation was like a red rag to a bull, more likely to escalate the self-harm than reduce it. It was hard to keep my mind present, so powerful was the pull to mentally turn away from what I was seeing. I also felt completely useless and, like the nurses at the hospital, dearly wished I could hand Sean on to a colleague for a while. Then, unexpectedly, something shifted. The following material came towards the end of a session when I'd had to keep telling Sean to stop doing various things which were dangerous or which he knew were not allowed.

Sean throws the ball into the air and makes a sideways dive. He lands on the floor with some force, banging his head lightly on the wall. I ask if he is okay. He says "stupid wall" and thumps it hard. I worry about his hand. He turns to look at me and gives me a ghastly, flirtatious smile. Still smiling, he flicks his head sideways and hits the wall with it. We look at each other. Sean hits his head against the wall again, this time a little harder. I say "ouch!". Sean's eyebrows shoot up and he looks at me with surprise. He hits the wall with his head again. I say "ouch" again but louder this time. Sean laughs and gets up. He goes over to his box, finds a marble, puts it into his mouth and pretends to swallow it. I tell him to spit it out and hold out a tissue. He spits it out then says "you passed the test, you're not stupid, let play the table football game".

The self-harm occurred when Sean felt he had disappointed or upset me. Previously, as described with the ball games, Sean controlled contact with me (and the fear of another failed attempt at attachment) by quickly moving away from direct one-to-one to solo activity. He then used the solo game to act out his profound belief that he was bound to fail.

In the clinical example above, it seemed as though Sean had moved from illustrating his fear of failed contact via the ball game, to experiencing it in the therapy room in relation to me. He felt he had failed to communicate his emotional state to me and was disappointed in himself. He then projected that disappointment into me and imagined I thought he'd let me down and was cross with him. The ensuing sense of failure and fear of retaliation Sean felt was overwhelming. He began to emotionally fragment and used his body to show me this was happening by, for example, hitting his head against the wall. The 'ouch' noise was experienced as an appropriate representation of his emotional state and bodily action. He felt understood and contained which led to a more cohesive internal state. Most importantly, we had found a way of relating to each other that Sean could tolerate and which was helpful.

It seemed crucial to think of Sean as a disturbed toddler in these moments, as an infant with no experience of maternal reverie (Bion, 1962) and, therefore, no benign internal means of self-soothing. This enabled me to find the appropriate means to acknowledge and validate his experience, thus helping him to make emotional sense of what was happening and providing the sense of containment which allowed him to put himself back together again. These 'ouch' moments were brief but significant. They involved noises and the odd word, but rarely sentences. The little boy emerging from the rubble was not used to the light, could only tolerate limited exposure and was going to need time to acclimatize.

My focus shifted increasingly towards trying to make sense of what Sean's body was telling me.

When I open the waiting room door to collect him, Sean does not look at me. The foster parents look exhausted and barely smile. Sean goes upstairs ahead of me and into the room without holding the door open. I enter and he is standing over his box. I sit in my chair. There is no eye contact from Sean. He picks the ball up and throws it hard against the wall. It ricochets across to the other wall. Sean ignores it. He walks towards the door and stands with his back to me. He then begins to walk around the room with a gangster gait. He is serious and deliberate. He sucks his teeth. After a few circuits of the room, I join him. I also adopt the gangster gait. We circle the room in silence for a few minutes. Sean then sits down. I also sit down. He leans forward in his chair, hands clasped in front of him and sighs. I say "tough week?" He nods with a world-weary expression, picks up the ball and throws it to me.

This body mirroring (Winnicott, 1971) seemed to develop out of the 'ouch' moments, as though we were building up a vocabulary of containment, adding movement to the sounds. It also became an important feature of the therapy. We began many sessions silently walking around the room. I would mirror what Sean was doing, using my body to convey an understanding of his state of mind. It was not like a dance or a reciprocal exchange. There was no eye contact. The connection was of two bodies moving in a similar way in time and space, as though we were tuning into each other, trying to find a wavelength we could share. Like the 'ouch', the mirroring became a way of letting Sean know that I understood something about how he felt, and in so doing, enabled him to make a link between his body and his emotional state. This allowed us to connect to each other in a way that was tolerable, using something external – the body – to share an understanding of something about Sean's internal life.

During the assessment period Sean had presented as polarized aspects of himself. As the therapy developed, a different kind of role play emerged.

> *We spend the next ten minutes playing cricket. Sean is very serious in his bowling, trying to copy professionals. A few times he cheats outrageously in blocking me from completing my runs. After one of these moments, when I point out that I have to be the loser at all costs, I bat and the ball hits Sean on the ear. The shot isn't hard and the ball is made of foam, but he clutches his ear and staggers dramatically. I take it very seriously and guide him towards the chair and sit him down. He says that since travelling on the aeroplane, every time he hits his ear it's really sore. He sounds like a much younger child and there is a whining, unfair tone in his voice. I get him to hold his nose and swallow, then to pretend to yawn and his ear eventually pops. I show him how to massage the back of his ear and it soon feels better.*

We were both role playing aspects of ourselves – Sean, hurt little boy, me concerned and kindly adult – and we both knew it, but it felt as though this was the only way we could be connected. I don't mean that it was a false interaction, on the contrary, it felt like a slightly theatrical version of a very authentic interaction. Because of the real intimacy involved it felt necessary to heighten or exaggerate the roles to create a safety net (that it was just a game) and to give Sean a sense of being in control of taking in something good.......a potentially dangerous move on his part. Again, this felt like a development or a 'moment of meeting' (Stern et al., 1998) – the ouch to the mirroring, then on to a heightened version of self.

We began to play out various scenes where Sean was hurt or in danger and I helped or saved him. Sean then began to bring imaginary friends into the play and to give me a more aggressive role.

> *Sean, still wrapped in the blanket, hides behind the chair, making himself small. He speaks to his imaginary friends "lets hide down here and then*

the blind, zombie witch won't find us." Then, to me, he whispers urgently "you be the witch looking for us, there's 2 boys and 3 girls". I sniff loudly. I say "I smell a boy" and pretend to look for him. As I search, between sniffs, I add more descriptions of what I can smell:
"I smell a boy who thinks he has to be strong and tough all the time
I smell a boy who has a sore knee
I smell a boy who doesn't get much sleep
I smell a boy who is good at grammar
I smell a boy who wants to have friends
I smell a boy who thinks people want to trick him so it's hard to trust anyone"
The feeling in the room changes to something gentler and calmer. I am close to Sean. I give him a chance to move to another hiding place (this is something he has done before) but he stays where he is wrapped in the blanket. He reaches through the gaps in the crocheted squares and gently touches my arm, then withdraws his hand. I squat down beside him. He reaches out his hand and takes my hand, like a little child. He reaches up and touches my face. I say he is touching my chin, cheeks, eyes etc. There is something tentative and gentle about his touch. He then takes my hand and uses it to touch his face. I say that I am feeling his eyes, chin etc and he can feel my fingertips on his face. There is a fragility about what is going on that makes me feel a little wary of what might come next, but there is no sabotaging act. He touches my neck and says "you're soft". It's time to finish. I say that it's time for us to tidy up. I stand up. Sean turns to his imaginary friend and says "I think your mum's here".

This session also felt like a turning point in the therapy. For the first time, Sean was able to trust it was okay to be little, curious and 'discoverable'. I started the game as a zombie-witch mother and ended it as a trusted maternal object. The space now felt safe enough to contain a vulnerable baby who wanted to be discovered and connected, rather than the perverse baby who wanted to sexualize, corrupt and control any attempt at contact.

It felt as though Sean was showing me what had happened to him, without words. Therapists sometimes refer to the therapy box as a representation of the patient's internal world. Sean's was in pieces; broken, fragmented and without a lid. His experiences of dying, coming back to life, the physically shocking experience of drug withdrawal, the perverse couplings and crushing humiliations he had suffered were all in his body. He used his body to show me his past and in mirroring his internal states, bearing silent witness to his experiences and working in role to allow him to safely explore his sense of self, I was able to help him process them.

The shared experience of shifting through the rubble of Sean's life created a therapeutic relationship based on trust and understanding.

Sean pulls out the green lego box and puts the round sellotape, with the ball balanced on it, under the box. He creates a wobble board and tells me that he is going to try to balance. He closes his eyes and mutters something under his breath. He works very hard and delicately to keep his balance. He says "can you stand here so that you can catch me if I fall?" I stand up and face him, so that I can steady him if he falls forwards. We look each other in the eye. Sean really concentrates. It feels as though he is using my eyes to maintain his balance. He knows I am ready to catch him if he wobbles and a few times I think he deliberately tips forwards to make sure I will react and steady him. This game lasts a long time and it is the calmest I have ever seen him.

Discussion

Sean, born out of the rubble of his mother's drug-ridden womb, had to fight for survival from the moment he was conceived. Having had no experience of maternal reverie, he had little capacity to recognize feelings or to process, reflect upon or learn from them. If the therapy room is a child's first opportunity for any kind of shift from a hypervigilant, reactive stance to a less persecuted more receptive state of mind, then the initial step must be to allow the patient the space and time to express what they have been through using whatever means they have at their disposal. When the trauma has happened before the child has developed language to describe their experience (and language belongs to the trauma-giver) it seems that the body retains the most accurate account of what they have been through. In rushing to attach words to this physical expression the therapist can unhelpfully miss out a stage in the child's therapeutic development, the stage which I describe as sifting through the rubble. Before helping the child to understand and attach meaning to what they have gone through, the therapist first needs to acknowledge and bear witness to what their experience has been. I believe this process, of slowly and safely making something conscious in the presence of another, without falling apart, is the preparation for the house building stage which Anna Freud describes. It is a process which cannot be rushed. As Melzer said "sometimes one needs to tiptoe up to the pain" (Donald Melzer, quoted in Boston & SZur, 1983).

Finally, I would like to speak about my clinical experience of sifting through the rubble. This process is different with each patient. It involves an adaptation of technique, but not always the same adaptation. It is vital that each patient is thought about as a unique individual (Horne, 2019). In this case it involved using my voice and body to convey an understanding of Sean's experiences. Noises were more containing than words. Mirroring and working in role became safe methods of creating authenticity in the interactions between us. When Sean arrived as a gangster and walked around the room, initially it felt as though he was trying to keep me away. When I joined him in this gangster state of mind and body, what started as a defensive state became a point of connection, a way of tuning into each other and creating a meaningful exchange. Seeing his own body state mirrored enabled Sean to make a link between his body and a feeling he was having, because I knew about it, could feel it and communicate it. This gave him a sense of containment and an experience of being emotionally in synch with another which felt safe and could be taken in. The emphasis was to facilitate Sean's acknowledgement of what had happened to him not, as this stage, to discuss why it happened or what the experience meant.

Sean and I continued to work together for several years. The therapy developed and we tentatively began to explore issues around 'why' as well as 'what'. We slowly added more language. This was not plain sailing. When things went wrong for Sean as they sometimes did, he would quickly revert to physical communication, as though the early trauma had been reactivated and a non-verbal, physically enacting default position taken up. I would alter my response accordingly and we would return to a more physical means of communication until Sean felt safe. The 'sifting through the rubble' process was not only the way into therapy for Sean and I, but has also gave us a safe place to return to when things went wrong. In this case, securing the danger zone, assessing the damage and sifting through the rubble brought about the possibility of a new internal structure being built with containment and understanding in the foundations and enough flexibility in the design to survive potential aftershocks.

I am very grateful to Anne Alvarez who supervised my work with Sean.

References

Alvarez, A. (2012) *The thinking heart: three levels of psychoanalytic therapy with disturbed children*. London and New York, Routledge.

Bion, W. R. (1962) *Learning from experience*. London, Heinemann. New York, Basic Books.

Boston, M. & Szur, R. (eds.) (1983) *Psychotherapy with severely deprived children*. Exeter, Karnac.

Campbell, D. (2005) Perversion – sadism and survival. In: Budd, S. & Rusbridger, R. (eds.) *Introducing psychoanalysis: essential themes and topics*. East Sussex and New York, Routledge.

Horne, A. (2019) *On children who privilege the body: reflections of an independent psychotherapist*. London and New York, Routledge.

Joseph, B. (1982) In: Spillius, E. B. & Feldman, M. (eds.) *Psychic equilibrium and psychic change: selected papers of Betty Joseph*. London, Routledge.

Morgan, D. (2007) Perverse patients' use of the body- their own and that of others. In: Morgan, D. & Ruszczynski, S. (eds.) *Lectures on violence, perversion and delinquency: the portman papers*. London, Karnac.

Sandler, J. Kennedy, H. & Tyson, R. (1980) *The technique of child psychoanalysis: discussions with Anna Freud.* London, Hogarth Press.

Stern, D., Sander,L., Nahum, J., Harrison, A., Lyons-Ruth, K., Morgan A., Bruschweiler-Stern, N., & Tronick, E. (1998) Non-interpretive mechanisms in psychoanalytic therapy: the "something more" than interpretation. *International Journal of Pscho-Analysis.* 79, 903–921.

Van der Kolk, B. (2014) *The body keeps the score: mind, brain and body in the transformation of trauma.* London and New York, Penguin Books.

Winnicott, D. W. (1964) Aspects of juvenile delinquency. In: Winnicott, D. W. (ed.) *The child, the family and the outside world.* England, Penguin Press.

Winnicott, D. W. (1971) *Playing and reality.* New York, Basic Books.

Chapter 11

Embracing darkness: clinical work with adolescents and young adults addicted to sexual enactments

Ariel Nathanson

This paper described common themes and transitions in the treatment of adolescents and young adults presenting as addicted to sexual enactments. Central to their experience is a highly addictive reliance on a bad object, which both enables and relies upon sexually perverse enactments. The paper follows the therapeutic process with patients seen in either group or individual long-term psychotherapy. Their experience is understood in the context of theories central to the work at the Portman Clinic relating to perversion and addiction, combined with some ideas from the field of criminology. Patients usually start by noticing their relationship with their compulsive behaviour, moving from a passive stance to a perception of themselves as active agents. They discover moments that are described as 'pressing a button', at which they move from passivity to taking perverse action. Those insights lead to a slowing down of the addictive cycle and emergence of phantasies, core complex anxieties and even hopes, all desperately avoided by taking sexualized action. The paper follows a pathway of change and transformation, which when successful enables patients to reduce or cease addictive behaviours by coming in contact with a good object, enabling both emotional pain and the experience of potency and hope.

Introduction

Owen, a young man in his third year of individual psychotherapy, described his need to give in to an addictive state of mind and enact sexually after being emotionally hurt by his girlfriend:

> *I hated what she did to me, hated her and hated myself for trusting her. I put some cuckolding porn on and spent hours masturbating to an idea of her betraying me with another man ... it was as if I needed to stir in some dark sex into my emotional pain, stir it in like a cordial, changing the colour and taste of what it used to be, which I could then enjoy drinking.*

The cordial – sexualizing the aggression and hatred into a sadomasochistic controlling formula – is both perverse and highly addictive. Once stirred in, it cannot be simply stirred out, so that emotional pain and sexual excitement remain connected as two inseparable molecules. Sustaining emotional pain without needing to sexualize it and enjoying sex without the habit of needing to stir pain into it both become extremely difficult to resist and highly addictive.

Bower et al. (2013) discuss many similarities between perversion and addiction, something I have noticed in all adolescents and young adults who are caught up in ritualistic cycles of sexual enactments that serve as a so-lution to core complex anxieties (Glasser, 1979), at times needing to triumph over or gain mastery over past sexual abuse. Glasser believed that the core complex is a universal conflict which is part of normal development in in-fancy. It is brought about in the context of early separation anxieties from the first attachment object, which induce a wish for a blissful fusion. However, being fused with the object creates a threat of engulfment and psychic annihilation. Those fears lead to hostility towards the engulfing object, which has now become a threat. There are two psychic alternatives to resolving this threat, both extremely anxiety-provoking; one is to destroy the object and the other to move away from it. Both of these solutions evoke what is referred to in this paper and elsewhere as core complex anxieties – the dread of destroying the object and the fear of abandonment and with-drawal from it. The perverse solution to this problem according to Glasser is the sexualization of the aggression towards the object, replacing the urge to attack the object with a sadomasochistic, ritualistic and sexually exciting controlling relationship. This solution allows for the expression of aggres-sion which is no longer a threat because it neither destroys the object nor creates a situation that would lead to abandonment. A very good example of this type of solution was a statement made by a patient, a young man who stopped being cruel to his girlfriend. He said, 'Now that I stopped hurting her so much I keep feeling anxious that she might leave me'. Indeed, like others, he did not feel anxious whilst he was being cruel and hurtful. Only when the sadistic control was no longer in operation did he feel the core complex anxiety he had attempted to keep at bay. The cordial, therefore, is a good metaphor for this sadomasochistic formula because it presents as a mind-altering substance which once consumed changes the way relation-ships are perceived and experienced (both to self and other). Writing in the same book, Wood (2013) shows that awareness and insight are never enough in propelling change in patients addicted to sex, and suggests that it can only occur once patients experience the anxieties at the basis of their addictions – the dreads that enactments protect them from.

Over the past few years, I have been working with many adolescents and young adults (all male) presenting with a variety of sexual addictions and other related harmful behaviours. During this time, I found that a few common themes and dynamics emerged in the work in quite similar ways. This paper is an attempt to map these themes, as they appear through the course of long-term psychotherapy, creating a pathway of development and change as patients struggle with their addictions, and begin to experience the anxieties their sexual enactments protect them from. I follow this process of change very closely and using my patients' descriptions and metaphors, offer some further insights into their experience of treatment.

Central to my patients' descriptions of their experience is an idea of descending into a dark world and their attachment to this dark landscape. The manner in which these young men spoke about darkness reminded me of the title and a specific section of a criminology book I read many years ago – *Salvation Through the Gutters*, by the Israeli sociologist and criminologist, Shoham (1979). The normative idea of salvation is quite similar to an oceanic phantasy state of union with a primary object; however, as I will show and discuss later, I believe that it has a darker version which is a state of union with a bad object rather than an ideal nourishing one. In his book Shoham analyses the mysticism of crime and social deviance. He conceptualizes the dynamic between subject and object as two opposing vectors: participation and separation. Deviant social behaviour, according to Shoham, is an attempt to 'neutralize' the normative social concept of being a separate human being. I think that neutralization of separation through deviance is quite similar to Glasser's idea of controlling the object through perversion. Shoham discusses his ideas in relation to mythology, culture and psychology. Amongst many examples, he quotes Jacob Frank, an eighteenth-century Jewish 'false Messiah' (i.e. falsely presenting himself as the long awaited for real Messiah), preaching to his followers:

> *I did not come into this world to lift you up but rather to cast you down to the bottom of the abyss. Further than this it is impossible to descend. The decent into the abyss requires not only the rejection of all religions and conventions, but also the commission of 'strange acts' and this in turn demands the voluntary abasement of one's own sense of self, so that libertinism and the achievement of that state of utter shamelessness leads to a state in which all laws and religions are annihilated.*

(*[Frank]*, Scholem, 1972:p.21) The idea of salvation through the gutters accurately captures my patients' experience of sex addiction, as they described it: a trigger facilitates a swift, at times unconscious pushing of a button that flips their world into a very familiar and soothing darkness. Darren, aged 17, described his addiction to pornography in the following way: 'It was the opposite of the false existence I had with my parents, the pretence that they were good and caring. In the dark I felt myself, my real self, not pretending, it always felt like the truth ... this was my real attachment ... my first love'. I think that this description is very similar to

Shoham's idea of the mysticism of evil. In psychological terms, it represents a mystical union with a bad object, highly addictive, giving rise to omnipotent and triumphant states of mind. It represents the perverse solution to the core complex described by Glasser (1979) because it triumphs over a need for a good object, protecting it from aggression and making abandonment irrelevant. This state of mind is much more than an identification with an aggressor (Freud, 1968). In fact, patients describe an experience of becoming part of something much bigger than themselves, triumphing over any abuse by nullifying it, inoculating themselves against any future or past pain in a world where love is hate and abuse is love, making sexual boundaries insignificant and crossing them as a way of showing allegiance and courage.

I believe that this is a sexually perverse incarnation of the internal gang described by Rosenfeld (1971), an organization resembling an internal cult, and that these patients are following a 'false messiah' by committing strange acts of sexual perversion as gestures of loyalty, directly challenging reality and the facts of life. The sadomasochistic cordial described by Owen, therefore, leads to a direct union with a cult-leader-bad-object offering sadomasochistic control of the core complex-inducing object and/or past and present abusers by changing the basic assumptions of the world they belong to and altering the laws of relationships.

The patients I will describe here are either in individual or in group therapy. They are presented with general background information which is typical to many Portman patients and therefore a direct link is never made between any one patient and a specific identifiable history. These patients initially present as suffering, highly addicted to their destructive activities and feeling at the mercy of those, unable to free themselves, as they would desperately like to do in order to lead a normal life. The first stage in their treatment reflects this specific presentation.

Passive suffering versus omnipotent triumph

Owen was referred aged 19 because of his propensity to erupt in violent rage in response to a variety of provocations, to hurt others and destroy property. He presented as depressed and lost, tormented by guilt, worried about his inability to control his violence, addicted to Internet pornography and at times actual destructive sexual encounters with strangers. Although a perpetrator of violence, Owen mainly presented as a passive suffering victim of his addiction and impulsivity. However, his excitement was soon expressed in his accounts of bizarre sexual encounters and pornographic imagery, presented with humour and excitement, as if inviting the listener to become a voyeur, sharing the images appearing in his descriptions or on Owen's computer screen and colluding with the excitement in laughing with his humour. Rather than depressingly describing his passivity, unable to control his behaviours and addiction, Owen presented a different image of his self, immersed in what he called his 'dark world', and derived a sense of intense pleasure in doing so.

Like other patients during this initial stage of treatment, Owen came to his sessions in a state of direct contact with the pleasure of his enactments and with the part of him that gained gratification from pain and triumphed over passivity, victimization and the impotent rage associated with them, all often accompanied by actual manic excitement. Effectively, as his therapist did not collude with the enactment, Owen started noticing his dual identity – the victim/perpetrator (Woods, 2003) – and how he seemed to always seek to avoid one state by being identified with the other.

A similar dynamic was very noticeable in my therapy group. As some patients spoke about their disturbing fantasies and actions with great shame and guilt, other patients, in parallel, secretly got excited by the narrative and imagery described. This was commented on by noticing with the group that whilst one of the members was describing his actions with great shame and pain in the group's 'front room', other members were secretly watching and masturbating to the images in the group's 'back room'. This interpretation, used in both individual and group settings, usually led to a reduction in the amount of pressure to enact in the sessions, and over time to patients noticing 'back room activity' and helpfully disclosing it in real time. The group became the embodiment of the abused/abuser identity, which could no longer be denied.

The internal cult

Becoming aware of his 'dark side', Ron, a 20-year-old patient addicted to masturbating to extreme sadomasochistic pornography, had a dream:

> He is lying on the floor of a public toilet, filthy, covered in excrement and urine. Surprised, he notices that he has an erection and starts masturbating, excited and feeling an intense sense of freedom.

Masturbating in the gutters clearly demonstrates how sexualization becomes an act of salvation in this underworld, showing loyalty and commitment to the internal cult, leading to the mystical union with the cult-leader/bad object. In the dream, the patient is initially terrified when he realizes where he is but quickly triumphs over his shock and disgust by masturbating to it. It is an attack on reality, an aspect of perversion highlighted by Limentani (1989) and others, confusing orifices, body functions and generational differences. It turns the potential disgust and claustrophobia into the necessary conditions for sexual excitement. The 'strange act', the perversion, frees the patient from the terrifying reality, in which he is both a victim and a perpetrator, turning it into an exciting, daring celebration.

This patient and others usually start noticing at this point that crossing boundaries is an act from which there is no return. Patients who act on their fantasies, those who harm others or masturbate to extreme imagery of any kind, are unable to forget or undo the commitment they have made through enactment, which they now describe as part of who they are.

Another patient, Garry, aged 21, was able to describe his journey into 'salvation' in the following way: since his early adolescence, he had felt inadequate and unworthy of girls' attention. He remembered very clearly being rejected by a girl when he was 13 and the humiliation and rage he felt. This was the time he started watching pornography, which became a refuge from these persecuting feelings. As he grew older, the sense of rejection and humiliation never stopped although he was actually quite popular and had real relationships with girls of his age. He identified a pattern that turned into a ritual: he would see a good-looking young woman in the street, look at her, feel inadequate, imagine her rejecting and humiliating him, hate her, fantasize about seeing her naked without her permission, go home quickly whilst already thinking about pornography, watch it, notice that it was not enough, not 'hitting the spot', escalate the content and eventually watch images of child abuse, which was the only thing that could end the ritual, a 'dose' high enough to triumph over the impotent rage. He would then feel full of shame, guilt and self-loathing. The addictive perversion here, as in all the other cases, served to encapsulate and manage the actual anxieties, which were hardly even glimpsed because even the memory of being humiliated aged 13 was probably just a screen memory masking much deeper phantasies and the anxieties attached to them. It allowed the patient to lead a normal life most of the time, only needing the cult at times of distress, when he felt threatened by the potential emergence of unconscious dreads.

This patient, like many others, reported experimenting with various enactments over many years until he reached the point at which his ritual was complete. Elaborating on Owen's metaphor, Garry had been unconsciously working for a long time on the exact formula for his specific sadomasochistic cordial, the code for a perfect perverse solution. I think that strange, perverse acts, such as the one he performed, should be seen as single-dose addiction makers. The salvation the patient experiences in the moment of action, immersed, excited, at one with the bad object, combined with the actual impact of the action and its severity, make it impossible to simply move away from. It is not a random act, like many patients present their first time. Rather, it is the end of an unconscious journey, a perverse eureka moment in which a match is found between a specific unconscious dread and the way to triumph over it.

The fuck-it button

This phrase, often used by many patients to describe a similar experience, refers to a very specific moment in time – the split second in which they move from passivity to action. Clinically, this has proved to be one of the most effective clinical concepts I use in working with these patients.

Exposing and understanding the button dynamic is often a turning point in treatment. Typically, as patients come to differentiate between a state of passive suffering, not wanting to act, and a state of active excitement and omnipotence, they are able to notice the moment of transition from one state to the other. Their narrative changes from a very passive 'giving into darkness' or being 'overpowered' to a single moment of active transition. Very significant to their treatment, patients are then able to notice which part of the self presses this button internally – noticing that it is they, the suffering patient in the therapy room that presses the button and actively invites in another part of their personality. Usually, the suffering patient then assumes the role of a collusive observer, repulsed by what he sees and excited by what he does. Strangely, patients often smile when this is noticed for the first time, surprised and often relieved or even excited to be found out. They discover, as a patient once said, that they are 'making a real active choice under extremely compelling conditions'.

Over time, some patients remember 'their first time' of pressing or even inventing this button, usually in the context of coping with actual ongoing traumatic relationships in childhood. Sexually abused patients, for example, typically describe a moment of taking the initiative, doing something the abuser was not expecting, trying to enhance his pleasure. This is remembered as a 'dare', a courageous act of crossing a boundary. In hindsight, as they analyse their current experiences of pressing this button in the context of their addictive cycles, they clearly notice how a single act transitioned them from passivity to taking charge, the moment they found salvation in the gutters.

Indeed, this powerful dynamic in childhood often severs the psychological link between body and mind and between factual memories of the past and the meaning assigned to them. The act of taking this initiative and taking charge distorts the reality of the trauma in a way that makes it inaccessible to reflection and thinking, giving rise to the common presentation in which patients take time to discover that they were abused, although remembering what had happened to them.

This dynamic is very clear in actual sexual abuse, but I do not think that it is specific to it. It can be a characteristic of other abusive and traumatic childhood experiences in which for a variety of reasons, a good object was unavailable and a bad object had to be conjured up instead. Under such traumatic circumstances, good objects are perceived (both internally and at times externally) to belong to the upper echelons of emotional life, a perfect relationship, unfitting of the gutters and threatened by darkness. The good object, therefore, is not there to flick a switch, turn on the light and claim the suffering child. In its absence, the terrified child flicks another button to induce an omnipotent state by turning to an object that seems to be always there, an object that distorts reality, marketing darkness as light and therefore making turning the light on unnecessary. Dependency on this object becomes a form of salvation in its capacity to convert abuse and trauma into something else.

I think that this dependency is by definition addictive because distorting reality requires repeated enactments in order to maintain and reinforce the distortion. It is the inversion of a relationship with a nourishing loving object which promotes the development of security and faith required for the perception of reality as it is and containing the emotional challenges it constantly evokes. A relationship with a good object harnesses the development that the cult thrives on perverting: the experience of separateness, separation and independence.

Significantly, as patients become aware of their reality-changing-button-pressing-moments, their narratives change and they are able to see, as if in slow motion, various aspects of their experiences before, during and after they press this button. They often feel more responsible for their actions and after a period of some excitement usually become increasingly depressed as they begin to notice the level of their addiction, and angry not being able to act differently.

Slowing down the ritualistic cycle

Becoming mindful of the button increases patients' awareness of other ritualistic aspects in their relationships to themselves and others. As a long-term group patient explained to a new member: 'It's not that you stop doing it … it just becomes really slow and you notice all the little things that happen, how you feel and then what you do'. Within this slowness of motion, patients begin to notice the various aspects of their enactments. The triggers are different and range from an inability to experience negative emotions in a benign way to the more extreme core complex anxieties or the need to triumph over past abuse and trauma. Other triggers are more circumstantial and specific, relating to the enactments themselves; the presence of a trigger image, a feeling, even a smell or the position of the sun on a winter afternoon, each can trigger a compulsion to act.

However, patients at this stage are able to notice these details and describe them because action cycles have slowed down. Indeed, the button is still pressed but during the time of thoughtful hesitation prior to letting go there are glimpses of both the anxieties that are being avoided and the potential for good experiences that had to be suspended or attacked.

Interestingly, the first part of the ritual to change in this destructive cycle is patients' levels of guilt and their perception of the damage they inflict in their enactments. I believe that the main reason for this is the realization that the guilt they feel at the end of their enactments is just part of the ritualistic cycle and not, as they initially present, something belonging to the actual aftermath.

As a result, instead of spending days or longer filled with masochistic punitive chunter (Joseph, 1982), often very suicidal patients describe a sense of being able to stay away from the ritual, experience some real emotional pain, real guilt, shame and loss, replacing the ritualistic masochistic version of these emotions. There is an acknowledgement of the full cycle, the choice made to enact, the need to do so and the actual damage that was inflicted.

Patients often notice at this point how they ritualize negative feelings as a way of mastering them, rather than face their anxiety about having real emotional experiences, unpredictable and unscripted. As a result, they begin to experience their enactments as 'clinical'. There is often some change in the content of enactments too, which becomes very specific, still self-destructive but not harmful to others. Patients now feel that they know what they are doing, acknowledge an emotional state that they cannot tolerate, press the button, act and emerge feeling that something has been evacuated. Feelings of emptiness, guilt and failure are then kept to a realistic minimum as patients become able to hold on to more complex narratives relating to their past, being mindful of links and less terrified of having feelings. Their grip of a bad object seems to be lessening as the potential for a good experience becomes more available. Although they are not free from enactments or addiction, this is a significant developmental move.

Mystical union versus separateness and integration

When patients become less addicted to the activities that symbolically and concretely maintain the mystical union with the bad object, they start to develop a sense of separateness. As they begin to tolerate this state for longer periods of time, they begin to evaluate some of their actual relationships to real others. Anger and assertive aggression begin to replace chronic resentment, apathy, sexualized hatred and pathological guilt.

One patient aged 15 at the beginning of treatment started his first assessment session with the following aggressive statement: 'I'm worried about you spoiling my relationship with my mother and I'm not going to let this happen'. Three years later, now free from his sex addiction and feeling separate from his highly intrusive smothering mother, he recalled his first statement in the first session and said, 'It's funny how furious I was with her then and didn't even know it ... I confessed my sexual sins to her, self-harmed and got her to take me to A&E every week instead. Now I get angry ... it's not too bad'.

With a lessening of the ritualistic predictability of sadomasochistic relationships, patients feel exposed to a spectrum of emotional experiences that were previously defended against. They struggle to find ways to experience negative feelings in a benign way. Anger is often very difficult to tolerate, together with jealousy, aggression and disappointment. Once they are able to experience some of those feelings without needing the cult's help, without 'mixing in the cordial', a long and painful period of emotional and relational instability ensues.

As separation and separateness become available as a potential, there is a resurgence of adolescent conflict and behaviour, which has never been worked through. The 15 year old described above, for example, was able to start annoying his parents, having conflict, worrying them, rather than heavily controlling them with the threat of suicide on the one hand and confessions of his sexual addiction on the other. Adolescence as a developmental force can be very helpful therapeutically as long as patients are helped to differentiate between the benign and the perverse, between aggression and hatred, anger and punitive control. These young patients often find the courage at this point to confront their parents or others for the first time, able to express a narrative of their childhood and have real questions that need answering. Some enact aggressively and even punitively but still within the remit of an adolescent developmental process rather than the ritualistic sadomasochistic cult practices. What they all seem to seek is an opportunity to experience separation and separateness rather than the need to control their objects, managing core complex anxieties or the actual implications of trauma and abuse.

Owen, for example, after four years of treatment, was able to differentiate between the abused and the abuser parts of his self. He said very simply: 'There is no balance between what I did to others and what was done to me ... no equilibrium'. Another patient, addicted to being physically smothered during sex, described a moment of change in the following way:

> I had a really bad day at work and I was on the bus home, calmly getting off on the porn that I was planning to look at when I got there. Then it was as if I was telling the group about it already, what I felt, how I pressed the button, what I did. I looked around me at all the other people on the bus, and as I was stepping out I saw a nice looking woman and smiled at her. She smiled back and suddenly I found it all so funny, I might have laughed out loud, it just felt so stupid. I then knew that I'd have something different to say in my session.

This patient's experience of 'looking around', seeing other people, meeting their eyes, being seen, smiling, the benign sense of life around him, was experienced in sharp contrast to his internal world, already geared up for perverse action. He then felt separate to the darkness, and the contrast was funny for him to experience. A good object was available in the form of his group, internally active in helping him perceive reality differently, observing and reflecting on his state of mind.

Emerging potency

Moments of not-pressing-the button and struggling with the results of no-enactments are eventually experienced as moments of potency. As most of these patients are sex addicts, not enacting means the end of constant masturbatory activity.

Clive, now 25, a group patient who had managed to stay out of his addictive cycle for the past two years, tried to explain the change he experienced. He said, 'We are all here because we do stuff. The most difficult thing in the world is to feel it coming and not act on it … to sit with it. It is like sitting with excruciating pain and not being able to touch it'. He returned to thinking about potency, a subject he was preoccupied with at the beginning of treatment. The potency he experienced then, through masturbation, was perverse because he enacted fantasies of abuse, using his penis to hurt others. He noticed over time that once he pressed the button he 'invited an abuser's hand to masturbate his penis', creating the excitement that would triumph over his tormented mind, his impotent rage and hatred of himself for not being able to stop the bullies who tormented him in the past. Clive could now notice the difference between omnipotence and potency, and how he needed an omnipotent triumph in order not to be at the mercy of his impotent rage and constant revenge fantasies.

As this process was slowed down and Clive became more thoughtful and able to tolerate more pain and non-masochistic guilt, he noticed how not enacting sexually made him feel more potent, creative and able to use his aggression to assert himself at work. However, he could also see how if the potency was left 'only in his body', as he phrased it, it became dangerous as if he could not experience it without it being attached to abuse. As the patient no longer used pornography, he had to actually experience this conflict and anxiety, which he now managed by returning to an old adolescent pattern of superficially cutting himself. In this context, the cutting was seen as development, trying to move on and do something different. It literally helped the patient to move away from his penis, therefore creating a potential for something else to happen.

Feeling less destructive, this patient found a girlfriend for the first time. He experienced being in love and enjoyed a sexual relationship that he completely split off from his other 'dark world', which was now experienced as under control and less needed. Although split off and somewhat equilibrated with past and present addictive processes, Clive enjoyed a sense of potency he never experienced before. Cutting was kept to a clinical minimum and Clive was not depressed. However, over time, being in a relationship evoked old core complex anxieties, now without the means to perversely manage them. Clive became paralysed whenever he felt angry. He would then either freeze, almost unable to move his body, feeling claustrophobic or literally have to run away, as far as possible from his girlfriend, in fear that he might hurt her. He did not know how to tell the difference between feeling angry, aggressive, assertive or violent. Any sense of anger would induce panic about what he might do in the same way that any erection seemed to point to abuse, which had to be masturbated away or contained by another physical addiction. Clive was eventually able to contain his anxieties and move on but sadly the relationship did not survive the turmoil. Nevertheless, he was able to painfully separate rather than go back to his addictive cycle.

In general, I have noticed that at this stage, the relational mess and real relational difficulties patients have give rise to experiences that were previously avoided. Patients fall in love, have non-perverse sex, sex which is not, as one patients said, 'masturbating with my girlfriend's vagina'. They also get hurt, jealous, angry and rejected. Turning points during this stage in treatment are often about noticing that something is not working in a relationship and painfully separating rather than 'mixing in the cordial', pressing the button and sexualizing the aggression, turning to sadomasochistic ritualized control as before.

Ending

The idea of ending becomes available for these patients when group processes (either in group or individual therapy) replace the need for the cult and patients notice that therapy is mostly used for safety. Owen, for example, used his therapy at this stage in order to look for the benign in his experiences, making sure that he was entitled to feel angry or even aggressive, that he was not being paranoid. In general, most patients hold on to their newly found sense of potency whilst still needing support in letting go of the addictive excitement of omnipotence and the triggers and challenges of impotent rage. Indeed, as this is actually a lifelong challenge, some patients might not be able to hold on to their achievements without many years of regular therapeutic work.

Central to the work, as discussed previously, is integration between the physiological and psychological, often reconfiguring the relationship between their bodies and their minds after many years of addiction and abuse. Interestingly, I have noticed how many patients reaching this stage of treatment start to positively enact it by becoming mindful of their nutrition or suddenly worried about 'damage done to their bodies'.

Darren, in the last months of treatment after seven years, noticed how he had not been eating well lately. He described an episode of drunkenness which was fuelled by him not eating for almost 12 hours before he went out with his friends. He remembered very clearly the moment of deciding to avoid having his dinner, recounting an omnipotent feeling of triumphing over his hunger. It was, as he put it, 'As if I filled myself up with my hunger rather than the food I could have had if I wanted to'. In the language of this paper, Darren reached out to a messianic bad object that marketed hunger as nourishment. He achieved a moment of salvation – triumphing over his body, needing no food, parents or therapy, deriving all his energy from the absence of a good nourishing experience. This was a familiar narrative in his treatment, recounted with a big sigh, 'feeling stupid', acutely aware that soon, as therapy ended, he would not be able to tell his therapist about it.

One of my therapy group members offered a very helpful metaphor during his ending phase. He said that he felt that therapy saved his life but 'Now, after three years, I have realised that this lifeboat will never actually reach the shore. It is for me to jump and see if I can swim and get there'. I think that this idea accurately describes the experience of ending, which cannot be achieved from a position of passivity. The ending phase leads to a point in which patients need to fully introject every last bit of responsibility they have delegated to the group and/or psychotherapist and then, without pressing a button, putting some faith in a newly discovered or acquired good object, take courage and jump.

Concluding remarks

Patients arrive into treatment feeling overwhelmed and confused, the unconscious ingredients of their early traumas mixed into the exciting, sado-masochistic sexualized action solutions they have developed in order to cope. The therapeutic discourse in group and individual sessions is therefore action related, starting with the detailed excited descriptions characteristic of the early stages of treatment and later moving on to noticing the absence of action and its impacts. As was presented here, enactment is a solution to cope with unbearable internal tension, core complex anxieties and the real early experience of abuse and neglect. Coming into contact with these takes time and requires a flexible therapeutic position. I would like to dedicate this last section to describe this position, which allows for the unfolding of the various themes and metaphors presented here.

Needing to know the details of 'what patients do' rather than just getting to know 'who they are' is central to the assessment and the unfolding treatment. It includes the concrete details of the enactment, which when looked at carefully, under a microscope, in the language of Owen's cordial metaphor, shows the molecular links between the sadomasochistic cordial and the initial trauma and/or core complex anxieties it was designed to mask and remove from thinking. Therapeutically, therefore, enactment is a very specific form of attack on linking because it attacks the capacity to think whilst simultaneously holding the code for restoring links and meaning. The fuck-it button is a good example to how this is expressed clinically: identifying the button makes a part of the patient more available for self-observation and alliance with the therapeutic work. However, it clearly shows how this observing part of the patient is also the one responsible for pressing the button and immersing themselves in addiction and perversion. It functions as a 'double agent', initially presenting as a passive victim whilst harbouring an active perpetrator or a deep-seated collusion with one. As such, it embodies the duality of the enactment itself – an attack on linking masking the ingredients needed for restoring integration and the capacity to think.

The technical meaning of this statement is that enactments are not only unavoidable but also essential for understanding patients' unconscious communication. The various metaphors and themes presented in this paper are the result of a therapeutic process that found meaning in enactments and placed them within a much wider psychological context.

Working with patients who constantly engage in action rather than thought requires a particular therapeutic stance. Group therapy has been invaluable in helping me develop this therapeutic position and the capacity to spot enactments and make them available to some inspection. Indeed, compared to the pressure of being alone with the enacting patient, it is less anxiety provoking to observe patients enact with each other in a group session. In fact, I came to notice that many of the interpretations I had made previously were themselves a form of an enactment. When patients enacted in sessions as a way of coping with their anxieties I responded by enacting a psychotherapeutic role as a way of coping with my collusion anxieties of being duped by the double agent aspect of the patient. The constant focus on spotting the enactment and resisting it stifled the session, leaving the patient alone and the therapist rigid within a defensive pseudo-therapeutic position. It led to interpreting the unconscious reasons for enactment too soon, as a defence against collusion, increasing anxiety rather than containing it. Being drawn in without noticing, on the other hand, could equally mask the unconscious anxiety and increased patients' hopelessness. Not surprisingly, this technical difficulty mirrors the familiar dynamic of the core complex – arid abandonment or engulfment, a claustrophobic–agoraphobic experience often present in sessions.

Working in this atmosphere of duality, as described above, with a double agent patient, it is impossible to sidestep moments of collusion or, at the other end of the spectrum, to avoid becoming punitive or rejecting. Over time, it is possible to take on a therapeutic stance that can wonder about these dynamics in real time or a bit later. This position usually leads to patients noticing that they are 'doing it again' in sessions rather than presenting with total avoidance or further going underground to avoid detection. Similarly, when the experienced group patient explains to a newcomer how what they say or do impacts the group, he conveys an instant offer of partnership (as opposed to collusion), taking a therapeutic position alongside the new patient, already presenting the group as an alternative to the 'cult', a dependency on a good object to supersede addiction, and a loving playful intercourse to replace the strict rules of perversion.

I believe that this way of working with enactments, inspecting them whilst accepting their inevitable impact, creates a very specific therapeutic culture both in individual and group therapy. With time, this culture becomes the antidote to the addictive cult because tolerating the enactments in sessions and inspecting them create the basis for tolerating the anxieties and trauma that they mask and distort. In fact, taking on the enactment makes it less of an attack on linking and more of a communication, akin to a dream, that needs to be understood to further development.

The patients I work with who manage to stay the course of long-term therapy are the ones who manage to accept this new culture, which internally represents restoring or a recreating faith in a good object. Indeed, they are also the ones who come into contact with the anxieties lying at the core of their attachment to the addictive cult. In fact, in the spirit of the dual processes presented here, the core complex, the victim/perpetrator, passivity and action, the double agent patient and the nature of the enactment itself, I think that the two processes are inseparable; a good object is needed in order to contain the anxieties previously managed by the cult, and experiencing these anxieties is the only way a good object can make itself known to the patient.

All of these patients walk a very narrow path, experiencing an 'addiction to near death' (Joseph, 1982), for long periods of their treatment. Working with them requires support and a culture that does not shy away from taking risk on and working with it. The Portman Clinic provides this culture and structure, still, even within an overall milieu that is increasingly risk-averse and procedurally driven. I regard it as a privilege to be working with this patient group in this way. My patients' capacity to change is sometimes truly inspirational, against all odds.

References

Bower, M., Hale, R. & Wood, H. (eds.) (2013) *Addictive states of mind*. London, Karnac.

Freud, A. (1968) *The ego and the mechanisms of defence*. London, Hogarth Press.

Glasser, M. (1979) Some aspects of the role of aggression in the perversions. In: Rosen, I. (ed.) *Sexual deviation*. 2nd ed. Oxford, Oxford University Press.

Joseph, B. (1982) Addiction to near death. *International Journal of Psycho-Analysis*. 63, 449–456 (IJP.063.0449A).

Limentani, A. (1989) Perversions: treatable and untreatable. In: *Between Freud and Klein: the psychoanalytic quest for knowledge and truth*. London, Free Association Books.

Rosenfeld, H. A. (1971) A clinical approach to the psychoanalytic theory of the life and death instincts: an investigation into the aggressive aspects of narcissism. *International Journal of Psycho-Analysis*. 52, 169–178 (IJP.052.0169A).

Scholem, G. (1972) Redemption through sin. In: *The Messianic idea in Judaism*. New York, Schocken Books.

Shoham, S. G. (1979) *Salvation through the gutters: deviance and transcendence.* Washington, DC, Hemisphere Publishing.

Wood, H. (2013) The nature of the addiction in "sex addiction" and paraphilias. In: Bower, M., Hale, R. & Wood, H. (eds.) *Addictive states of mind.* London, Karnac.

Woods, J. (2003) *Boys who have abused: psychoanalytic psychotherapy with victim/ perpetrators of sexual abuse.* London, Jessica Kingsley.

Chapter 12

The history of the Portman Clinic

Marianne Parsons

The clinicians

1930s–1960s

The Portman Clinic has its roots in what was first called the Psychopathic Clinic, founded in 1931, and renamed the Institute for the Scientific Treatment of Delinquency (I.S.T.D.) in 1932. Grace Pailthorpe, a psychoanalyst, psychiatrist and surgeon, who had run a field hospital in World War I and then worked in prisons in Birmingham and Holloway, developed an attitude towards delinquency that favoured treatment over punishment. Inspired by her research and ideas, other psychoanalysts, principally Dr Edward Glover, Dr Kate Friedlander, Dr Marjorie Franklin and Dr David Eder, set up a clinic with charitable status specifically to try to learn more about delinquency.

The I.S.T.D. accepted referrals of patients of all ages, the majority of whom were adults, but quite a number of children and adolescents were seen from the start. Initially, patients were seen in the analyst's own consulting room until a room for the clinic was secured in the mid 1930s at the Western Hospital, then it found its own first home in Portman Street in central London. With the establishment of the NHS in 1948, the clinical arm of the I.S.T.D. separated from its parent organization to become the Portman Clinic and part of the NHS, though the two organizations continued to share the building until the Clinic moved to its current location in NW3 in 1970 (Fishman & Ruszczynski, 2007).

Edward Glover spearheaded the clinical arm of the I.S.T.D. and so can be given the honorary title of 'the father of the Portman Clinic'. A staunch Freudian, he wrote two classic books that drew on his work there – The Early Development of the Mind (1956) and The Roots of Crime (1960). Glover always emphasized the importance of a careful diagnosis so that appropriate recommendations could be made, and this is as important now and it was then. For many years, the Portman held an annual Glover lecture in honour of its chief founder. Kate Friedlander, a colleague of Anna Freud, was influenced by August Aichorn's work in Vienna with difficult adolescents and her main interest was in juvenile delinquency with an emphasis on both psychological and social therapeutic measures. In her book The Psychoanalytic Approach to Juvenile Delinquency (1947) she described her formulation about the origins of delinquent behaviour, namely a neglectful and negative environment that threw off course a normative development process and led to a weak ego and undeveloped superego unable to 'modify strong drives for pleasure seeking' (Nolleke, 2019). Marjorie Franklin developed an early interest in the relationship between mental illness and the patient's environment and developed a therapeutic concept called 'Planned Environment Therapy' (PET) that she tried out at the so-called Q Camps for maladjusted young men and boys in 1930s–1940s. 'According to this milieu-therapy, theoretically inspired by Winnicott, Anna Freud, Otto Shaw and I. D. Sutie, patients live in a therapeutic community ... treated by a psycho-analytically supervised staff team' where they were encouraged to establish 'non-authoritarian, loving and accepting relationships' (Nolleke, 2019). Several male adolescents were referred from the I.S.T.D. to these camps. David Eder (credited by Freud as the first practising psychoanalyst in England, one of the founders of the London Psycho-Analytical Society and a founder member of the London Labour Party) always attempted to relate psychoanalytic thinking to political issues. He worked publicly for social reform and justice in general, but particularly with regard to the needs and care of children, women and what were then called 'mental defectives' (Thomson, 2011).

Within a short time, other psychoanalysts joined the I.S.T.D. clinic: Dr Wilfrid Bion, Dennis Carroll, Dr Aubrey Lewis, Barbara Low, Dr John Rickman, Dr Melitta Schmideberg, Karin and Adrian Stephen and Dr Sybille Yates. They were all inspired by a social conscience and an acute awareness of the very poor child welfare conditions at the time, especially amongst working-class families. Some had worked with young people but, as there was then no formal child and adolescent psychotherapy training, those who saw young people at the clinic gained further clinical experience by 'learning on the job'.

One of the most celebrated and well-known clinicians who worked with children and adolescents at the I.S.T.D. was John Bowlby, but he was unable to stay long and had to leave the Clinic when he was called up for World War II in 1940. Then there was Emmanuel Miller, father of the theatre director Jonathan Miller. He has been called the 'father of British child psychiatry' – the others given this honorary title were Donald Winnicott and Michael Rutter. Emmanuel Miller founded the first child guidance clinic in the East End of London in 1926 and in the 1930s took several I.S.T.D. child and adolescent cases in therapy at the West End Hospital for Nervous Diseases and the Maudsley Hospital. There was also Marion (Mollie) Mackenzie who had worked with Winnicott at the

Paddington Green clinic. She was inspired by him to work with children and later worked with John Bowlby at the Tavistock Clinic (Goldsmith, 2000).

In the 1950s–1960s, there was Herta Graz (a colleague of Anna Freud) and William Paterson Brown (who gained a fellowship in child guidance at the London Child Guidance Clinic), both of whom were long-standing members of staff and saw a huge number of young people at the Clinic, and Henry Dugmore Hunter who later set up the adolescent unit at the Tavistock Clinic. There was also the wonderfully eccentric Josephine Lomax Simpson who founded centres in Wimbledon in the 1970s for single young mothers and their babies as well as homeless young men, where her provision of Smarties as a substitute for anti-depressants was dubbed by Private Eye as her 'therapeutic Smartie technique'! (Rodway, 1999). Over the years, other adult psychoanalysts also treated older adolescents/young people at the Clinic, including Wilfrid Bion, Michael Fordham, William Gillespie, Adam Limentani, John Rickman, Ismond Rosen and Lothair Rubinstein.

1970s–1980s

Phyllis Tyson (trained under Anna Freud at the Hampstead Clinic) was the first qualified child and adolescent psychotherapist to join the staff. Many years later, she and her husband Bob Tyson wrote to my mind one of the best and most comprehensive books on development (Tyson & Tyson, 1990). Don Campbell (also trained at the Hampstead Clinic) took over her sessions in 1973 and became a very influential and long-standing member of staff who accrued a vast amount of experience with forensic patients during his 31 years at the Clinic, where he also was Chairman in the early 1990s. After qualifying as an adult psychoanalyst in 1976, he saw mostly adult patients at the Clinic, but he did work with some adolescents and he supervised all later child and adolescent psychotherapists on the staff even after he retired in 2004. His experience of working with adolescents at the Portman Clinic has informed his writing about violence, suicide and paedophilia. Two papers about adolescence stand out: 'Charles: a fetishistic solution' (Campbell, 1989) about an adolescent he treated at the Brent Consultation Centre, a walk-in centre offering assessment and analysis for adolescents in crisis (Laufer & Laufer, 1989Laufer 1989), and 'Breaching the shame shield: thoughts on the assessment of adolescent child sexual abusers' (Campbell, 1994), which describes how internal conflicts intensified by puberty and adolescence contribute to sexually abusive behaviour.

Dr Mervin Glasser, an adult psychoanalyst who joined the staff in 1971, became a very significant figure in the history of the Portman Clinic and was Chairman twice. Although not trained to work with children or adolescents, he was very keen to develop child psychotherapy at the Clinic. He was still working at that time at the Brent Consultation Centre where he undertook some analytic work with late adolescents and, together with colleagues, developed ideas about self-harm and suicide (Friedman et al., 1972). He set up a Violence Research Workshop at the Portman, which he spearheaded until his death in 1993. Although most of the patients studied in the Violence Research Workshop were adults, some adolescents were included when Dr Nicholas Temple joined the group. Giving very detailed attention to the session notes of their violent patients, the group studied the violent act, its immediate triggers and the background history of the patients. Over time they discovered that at the root of violence were severe developmental disturbances in narcissism (especially phallic narcissism), with the concomitant tendencies towards excruciating feelings of shame and humiliation. It was from this work that Mervin Glasser began to develop his concept of the Core Complex (Glasser, 1986, 1992, 1996, 1998), which is increasingly taking its rightful place in the body of psychoanalytic theory (see Chapter 1).

Don Campbell was the only qualified child and adolescent psychotherapist on the staff until Michael Morice (trained at the Tavistock Clinic) was appointed. In 1979, Dr Nicholas Temple, a psychoanalyst and child and adolescent psychiatrist, was appointed by Glasser specifically to work with adolescents. He soon set up the Adolescence Workshop with Michael Morice and Jeannie Milligan (social worker) as key members. Using his previous experience of working at the Cassel Hospital, Nicholas Temple introduced the use of family work, recognizing that disturbance in the family was often projected onto the young person. They developed a strong lively team taking many referrals, and the work with adolescents flourished. In 1983, they presented their clinical work at a very successful conference in Finland – it's a great loss to us now that they didn't publish their papers. Other staff members, who occasionally worked with an older adolescent or with parents, sometimes joined the Adolescence Workshop, including Don Campbell and Richard Davies, then a social worker, who later trained as a psychotherapist and was Director of the Portman Clinic from 2000 to 2005. Few children were seen at this time, mostly adolescents of 16 years or above: violent and delinquent patients (including quite a number of arsonists), many in turmoil about their sexual identity and with highly conflicted attitudes towards their bodies, and some potentially heading towards developing a full perverse structure.

1990s–2000s

When Michael Morice left the Clinic in 1984, Ora Dresner (trained at the Tavistock Clinic) was appointed. When she left, I took over from her in 1989 (having trained at the Hampstead Clinic, later renamed the Anna Freud Centre). As was the custom, I was given a month or two before seeing patients in which to settle into the Clinic by reading papers by Portman staff (past and present), looking through patients' files, and attending the Adolescence

Workshop and the weekly clinical meetings where a staff member would present a case. It felt very daunting to join such an illustrious psychoanalytic clinic, but it was also very exciting and stimulating, especially when I joined the Violence Workshop where Mervin Glasser was refining his ideas about the difference between sadistic and self-preservative aggression. To take part when he was developing his Core Complex theories in discussion with Don Campbell and the other group members was an enormous privilege. Using the model of Anna Freud's Diagnostic Profile with its emphasis on detailed exploration of a patient's development and metapsychology (Freud, 1965), we developed the 'Violence Portrait' to try to get an in-depth understanding of the internal world of the violent patients in the study. I remember the excitement when we discovered that every male violent patient in the study had erupted with self-preservative murderous violence when their defensive sado-masochistic way of relating broke down, and that the 'trigger' invariably concerned a perceived humiliating assault on their masculinity, i.e. their extremely vulnerable phallic narcissism. The unbearable humiliation resulted in their attacking the same part of the other's body that they felt had 'attacked' them, for example, the eyes that mocked them as small and weak, or the throat from whence came the verbal slight for being a 'mummy's boy'. Over time, several papers came out of this research: (Glasser , 1992, 1996, 1998; Campbell, 1994; Parsons & Dermen, 1999; Parsons, 2009, 2011).

In 1994, it became possible to increase the number of child and adolescent psychotherapy sessions. We were joined by Ann Horne (trained at the British Association of Psychotherapists, now renamed the Independent Psychoanalytic Child and Adolescent Psychotherapy Association – IPCAPA- at the BPF), for the first time making a team of three child and adolescent psychotherapists. Ann has drawn beautifully on her experience with Portman patients in her many writings (see the references section), which are full of sensitivity, wisdom and creative ways of engaging with children who are extremely hard to reach. John Woods (trained at the Institute of Child Psychology) was appointed in 2000, increasing the team to 4. When Don Campbell and Ann Horne retired from the clinic in 2004, Janine Sternberg and Valli Kohon (both trained at the Tavistock Clinic) were appointed.

Ariel Nathanson (trained at the Tavistock Clinic) joined the team in 2009. As a historical anecdote related to the Portman, he had worked at the Emmanuel Miller Centre, the same first child guidance clinic mentioned earlier. Shortly after he joined the Portman, NHS funding cuts reached the clinic and for the first time in many years, maybe even since its inception, clinical sessions had to be reduced. As a result, Janine Sternberg, John Woods and Valli Kohon had to reduce some of their work and take early partial or full retirement. Ariel Nathanson took over as referrals co-ordinator and for a long while was the only child and adolescent psychotherapist in the team still able to take on long-term work. A few years later, some funding became available even under this constant culture of financial cuts and instability, which continues today. The team started growing again: Patricia Allan (trained at the Tavistock) joined first, then Graham Music (trained at the Tavistock where he set up a training in psychotherapy & counselling) who writes widely on issues integrating body states with psychotherapeutic work and thinking. Tim Baker, (trained at the Tavistock) joined the team in 2018 when the Portman Clinic won a bid to set up a Forensic CAMHS service to consult to 13 boroughs in London. As a result, the Clinic became the host of a multidisciplinary team operating in a different culture but extending consultation work beyond its usual para-meters, making it available to many other children, families and profes-sionals. Another innovation was the creation of child psychotherapy training posts at the clinic. The first trainee was Eliza Newell who later joined the staff, the second was Cecilia d'Alancon, and a year ago the newest trainee, Marion Sangster, commenced her training post.

A comparison of child and adolescent patients referred from 1933 to the current day

Very fortunately, we can draw on a database spreadsheet compiled in 2018 from patients' files in the Portman archives from 1933 to 1960, which are now held by the Wellcome Trust (Amy Proctor, London Metropolitan Archives). I chose to focus on two different groups: the first 250 of all re-ferrals from the first patient in 1933 to the 250th in 1937 and the final 250 patients listed on the database in 1960. From these two sets of 250 patients, I extrapolated the children and adolescents so as to give some idea of young patients seen in the 1930s and 1960s and to which I could add some mem-ories of my own when I worked at the Clinic in the 1990s. This would then give impressions of three decades of work with children and adolescents, each 30 years' apart.

The 1930s and 1960 Portman Clinic data are divided into 5 age groups: under 10 years of age, 11–13 years, 14–16 years, 17–19 years and 20–21 years. From the beginning, as now, referrals of children and adolescents were dealt with in a number of different ways: consultation only to the re-ferrer/organization, report only (for the Court or Probation Service), as-sessment interviews with the patient, help for the parents/carers, recommendation for change of placement, school, etc. and/or offer of psy-chotherapy. There were several youngsters, particularly in the data from 1933 to 1937, who ran away from home, children's homes or hostels and who were often brought before the court 'in need of care and protection'. The frequent recommendation for a change of environment illustrates the clinicians' recognition of the traumatic impact of a deleterious external en-vironment on the child's development and well-being.

The 1930s

The wording and content taken from the Archive files between 1933 and 1937 is illuminating, and there are some very sad stories that reflect the attitudes and socio-economic conditions at the time. It wasn't uncommon in those days for children to leave school by or before the age of 14, and many of this age were described as 'unemployed'. This is a stark reminder of the hard times when many children had no ongoing education and little chance to get paid work when they left school.

Of the first 10 patients referred to the I.S.T.D. in 1933, half were aged between 14 and 18 years. The first two patients were both adults, but the third was an unemployed young man of 18 diagnosed with religious mania who was charged with fraud for 'taking expenses when impersonating a preacher'. He was offered therapy with David Eder, but there is nothing in the notes that says whether he took this up or not. We would now describe him as an adolescent, but at the time he was most likely perceived as an adult. However, the 4th patient would then have been considered an adolescent. This was a 14-year-old schoolgirl who was 'difficult to manage'. The clinician listed against her name is Bion, though she was not actually seen at the Clinic, having been previously diagnosed as 'mentally deficient and unsuitable for treatment'. Today, a patient with learning difficulties would not necessarily be deemed unsuitable for therapy. The 6th patient was a 16 year-old boy who had stolen from his family, and the 7th was a 17-year-old boy who had been charged with two counts of delinquency (no detail given). Marjorie Franklin recommended admission to a camp for maladjusted boys where they would receive 'milieu-therapy'. Because of the limited nature of the recorded data, it is difficult to ascertain accurately which child or adolescent patient was the first one to take up the offer of psychotherapy, but it is likely to have been the 10th patient referred to the I.S.T.D., an 'illegitimate' 16-year-old girl who was initially adopted but living in a children's home at the time of referral. Her 'crime' is listed as 'wandering' as she frequently ran away from the children's home, 'getting into trouble with the police for it'. Sybille Yates, a psycho-analyst and psychiatrist with a special interest in child and adolescent development who saw several of the adolescent cases, noted this patient's 'depressed states associated with menstrual difficulties'. Therapy only lasted for six sessions as the girl gained employment as a hospital maid, only a year later to run away again and then be 'certified insane'. Perhaps she had an incipient psychosis, but she would surely have been traumatized by being abandoned both by her birth mother and then her adoptive parents. There may well have been a link between the depression associated with her 'menstrual difficulties' and reaching an age when she could become pregnant, perhaps at a similar age to when her unmarried mother gave birth to her, thus the identificatory possibility of repeating her mother's history could have been significant in the extent of her disturbance.

Only two children aged 10 years or under were referred between 1933 and 1937. In the 11–13 years age group, five girls and six boys were referred. Of the girls, two were referred for violence, two for truancy and one for whom there are no details except that she was referred on to the Child Guidance Clinic and made 'excellent progress'. Of the boys, five were referred for stealing, one for being 'peculiar, secretive, unstable and out of control' and one 13 year old for unspecified 'sexual offences'. The largest referral group (41%) was the 14–16-years-olds (15 girls and 24 boys), followed by the 17–19-year-olds where there were far more boys than girls (20 and 7, respectively), and in the 20–21-year-olds, there was an even number of 7 female and 7 male patients. In all these mid-late adolescent age groups, delinquency was the most common reason for referral. Of the adolescent boys referred, few took up the offer of therapy at the Clinic but several were referred on to the Q Camps set up by Marjorie Franklin.

Cases referred for delinquent behaviour 1933–1937

Much of the following material drawn from these early years, though fascinating, is very tantalizing as the notes on the database are often very brief, leaving many answerable questions. As the clinic was originally set up to study and treat delinquency, it isn't surprising that over half (62%) of the child and adolescent referrals concerned delinquent behaviour. This mostly involved stealing, shoplifting and truancy, but I've included 'running away' and 'behaviour problems' in this category. 'Out of control' was a frequent referral symptom, and some young patients were described as having 'a lack of a sense of responsibility'. It is informative, but also very sad, when we look more closely at the database: a few youngsters were referred for 'being dirty in (their) habits', a 15-year-old schoolboy was remanded for stealing a quart bottle of milk, and a 12-year-old schoolboy was put on probation for stealing cabbages. This brings poignantly to mind the poverty amongst working-class families in London in the 1930s as well as the strong arm of the law in those days for petty theft. But there is one story that touches the heart in a different way. This is of a schoolboy (his age is not given) who was referred by his headmaster for stealing money from other schoolboys. He was assessed as 'unstable, neurotic in reaction to (his) attitude towards his parents' by B.W. Crowhurst Archer, a psychiatrist who saw a large number of the youngsters referred to the clinic. The patient was referred on for individual treatment at the Child Guidance Unit at West End Hospital for Nervous Diseases where he was treated by Emmanuel Miller. There was a 'definite improvement' in him, but the treatment had to end because the boy's family could not afford the fares for him to attend. However, it states later, 'Headmaster paying fees to attend treatment'. Hooray for such a good-hearted headmaster!

Two children aged 10 years or under were referred for delinquency: an 8-year-old girl for 'pilfering' and a 9-year-old boy for truancy, vandalism, stealing and breaking and entering where the recommendation was for a better foster placement and change of school. In the 11–13-years age group, truancy was the most frequent referral reason for girls and for the boys it was stealing. In all later age groups, stealing was the most common form of delinquency for both boys and girls, with the addition of housebreaking, fraud and forgery for the older male adolescents. One 18-year-old boy arrested for housebreaking had been 'boarded out since a baby' with a 'history of alternating between foster parents and biological parents' and had been sent at 11 years of age to an approved school because he was 'beyond control'. It's good to see that this young man, with a background that was so disruptive and that probably left him feeling not wanted by anyone, was given therapy.

Problems with sexuality 1933–1937

Totally, 13.7% of the adolescents referred had problematic sexual urges and all were boys. The youngest, aged 13, had been expelled from school for unspecified 'sexual offences'. This is the first recorded case of sexually abusive behaviour in the database, but later there were five 14–16-year-olds, six 17–19-year-olds and one 20-year-old referred because of sexual offences (including indecent exposure, working as a male prostitute, gross indecency with a man, sexual abuse of a sister, and homosexuality). It needs to be remembered here that until 1967 homosexuality was illegal under the Sexual Offences Act. It was recommended that a few of these adolescents needed to be in a more conducive environment and about half had therapy. One 20-year-old had been resorting to many different bodily enactments. He suffered from 'periods of serious depression and nerves' and had 'difficulties with sexual desires, particularly masturbation', but he had been charged as well with taking and driving away a car and attempted shop breaking. Unfortunately, no details are recorded about his background, but it's good to see that he was one of those who had therapy.

Violence 1933–1937

In total, 11.6% of the children and adolescents were referred for violence. In those aged 11–13 years, there were just two girls: one for assaulting a 2-year-old and one for attacking other children. Amongst the 14–16-year-olds, there were two girls simply described as violent or having outbursts of temper, and three boys where the most serious assault was by a boy who attacked his father with a pair of scissors. There was one girl in the 17–19-year age group with 'violent outbursts', and two boys (one who seriously assaulted his mother and sister, and another who attacked two boys with a knife). Of the 20–21-year-olds, there was just one young woman whose mother had died when she was 3, and at 5 she'd been sent from abroad to a convent in England. When she was 17, she went to live with her father who 'attempted incest'. She tried to poison him, then attacked him with an axe. She had about 2 years of psychotherapy with Dennis Carroll. Very few others took up the offer of therapy – either they did not attend if therapy was offered or they were sent to remand homes or prison. It's hard to know why there were more girls referred for violence, when in later years the large majority of violent patients were boys. Could it be that a violent girl was seen then as much more disturbed and that male violence was more socially expected and tolerated?

1960

Looking at the last 250 of all referrals in the database, it is very striking to see how much the Clinic had grown in the previous 30 years. To remind us, the first 250 referrals to the I.S.T.D. had covered a span of four years, whereas the last 250 on the database were in one single year, 1960. So, the total number of referrals had leapt hugely, probably due to the fact that there had been a large increase in the number of staff and hours available to see patients. Administrative staff members had been employed to help with the running of the clinic and clinicians were now paid, whereas at the beginning, the clinicians worked for free and so had far less time to be able to see I.S.T.D. patients alongside maintaining their private practice. Importantly, by this time the Clinic was more widely known as a valued resource for referring very troubling patients.

I won't go into as much detail in this section as with the data from 1933 to 1937, largely because less detail was recorded, but will just point out anything that feels particularly significant in the data from 1960 compared with that in the 1930s. The most significant change was that the percentage of children and adolescents referred had risen from 38% to 57.6% of the total of all referrals. There was a similar percentage of children and adolescents of each sex in each age group as well as a striking similarity regarding the number of cases of delinquency (55.3% from 1933 to 1937 and 55.5% in 1960). There were fewer violent youngsters seen (down to 4.2% from 9.6%), but an increase in the referrals of young people with sexuality problems (up from 15.9% to 21.5%). And there were differences in outcome following assessment: there were fewer recommendations for a change of environment (down from 25.5% to 11.8%), and a healthy increase in patients taking up the offer therapy (up from 25.5% to 38.9%).

The 1990s

As the database ends at 1960, the following section draws on my memories of working at the Clinic in the 1990s. I recall we saw mostly male adolescents, but there were also quite a number of girls, as well as pubertal and younger children of both sexes. Several had been involved in incest with a sibling or stepsibling, and each young person in the incest pair then had therapy at the clinic. I remember a girl of 9, sexually abused by her stepbrother, who came dressed by her mother in revealing clothes looking like a seductive teenager. Her mother had been sexually abused herself as a child – a mother unwittingly offering up her daughter for abuse (due to identification with the aggressor as an unconscious defence against unbearable humiliation and shame), was something we were always alert to and made sensitively handled parent work vital. I recall a 12-year-old girl surprising me with her insight when she volunteered her confusion that her teenage brother was getting all the hostility for the incest: 'It isn't fair. I wanted it too'.

We treated many delinquent and violent youngsters, some with perverse behaviours (I saw a boy with a shoe fetish), and several who had sexually abused younger children. One sexual abuser comes to mind particularly as he illustrates the pervasive sense of shame that can act as a severe resistance in therapy. He was eventually able to express deep remorse and guilt about having abused two very young girls in an especially cruel way, but it took him many months to overcome his deep shame to be able to talk about having been sexually abused by his uncle. As the psychoanalyst Clifford Yorke said, 'Guilt can bring material into therapy, but shame keeps it out' (personal communication).

Child and adolescent psychotherapists at the Portman took on a number of tasks in the 1990s, as they still do: assessing and treating patients, work with parents and sometimes with families, court reports, consultations to the patient's network as well as to various institutions (such as Youth Offending Teams, children's homes), providing supervision (e.g. for social workers, child and adolescent psychotherapists in other settings, and adult-trained Portman staff seeing adolescents), and giving presentations and teaching in a wide range of settings. Some of us taught clinical seminars on forensic issues for child and adolescent psychotherapy trainings and we all taught on and/ or supervised students on the Portman Clinic Diploma in Forensic Psychotherapeutic Studies, of which I was course director from 2000 to 2008. In 2008, I retired after 19 years at the Portman, feeling very privileged to have learned an enormous amount from the patients and to have worked with so many inspiring colleagues; but few of us ever leave the Portman entirely! Several of us who are now retired from the Clinic continue to teach or supervise on Portman courses, and it's very good to hear that the Child Team at the Portman is continuing to flourish and that psychotherapeutic work with very vulnerable and traumatized child and adolescent patients is as valued by the rest of the staff as it was when I worked there.

The 2000s

There are two main differences between referrals during the 2000s and the previous decades. The first is the increased prevalence of the Internet, the arrival of smart phones, online social communication platforms and, in 2007, the arrival of free pornography. Young patients today have a portal to images of pornography and violence of the most extreme kind in their pockets. This is crucial in putting the idea of enactment within this chapter's historical context. The smartphone in the pocket can be a ready-made instant gateway into enactment. Seconds can pass between the introduction of a sexual thought in the mind to enacting it physically whilst watching something on the screen or using it to communicate disturbingly with others. The referrals reflect this change. In an audit of 86 patients referred in 2013/14 conducted by Patricia Allan, 84% were for difficulties of a sexually harmful nature and 16% for violence. The Clinic now treats patients with 'pornography addiction' and those who offend by looking at images of child sexual abuse on the internet. These enactments and offences were never so common and, as some chapters in this book will indicate, are facilitated and even caused by the availability of the internet.

The second difference between today's referrals from those of the past is the economic environment of the last decade following the financial crisis of 2008. This was and still is a time of austerity and drastic financial cuts to public services, especially NHS child mental health services, social care, education, the police and judiciary. This led to enormous gaps in services available to those presenting with psychological difficulties, and especially patients like those seen at the Portman who often require a network of various professionals cooperating in the care of one child.

Children and adolescents enact their difficulties because they did not get what they needed when they needed it. If we want to reduce risk, therefore, we need a system where risky children are not only restrained but also given the opportunity to get what they need in order to enable them to harness natural development towards positive change. When resources are very scarce, the little that services have is invested in managing risk by restrictions or by a variety of organizational defences psychologically designed to deny reality and turn a blind eye to the full picture. Child psychotherapists at the Portman are often in a position, maybe similar to their historical colleagues, of pointing out needs and deprivations without the means to address those and repair damage caused by trauma, as the state slowly withdraws its responsibility for providing adequate medical and social care to its citizens.

References

Campbell, D. (1989) Charles: a fetishistic solution. In: Laufer, M. & Laufer, M. E. (eds.)*Developmental breakdown and psychoanalytic treatment in adolescence: clinical studies*. New Haven and London, Yale University Press.

Campbell, D. (1994) Breaching the shame shield: thoughts on the assessment of adolescent child sexual abusers. *Journal of Child Psychotherapy*. 20 (3), 309–326.

Campbell, D. (2011) The nature and function of aggression. In: Williams, P. (ed.) *Aggression: from fantasy to action*. London, Karnac Books. pp. 1–15.

Campbell, D. (2014) Debt, shame and violence in adolescence: reactions to the absent father in the film bullet boy. *The International Journal of Psychoanalysis*. 95 (5), 1011–1020.

Fishman, C. and Ruszczynski, R. (2007) The Portman Clinic – an historical sketch. In: Morgan, D. & Ruszczynski, S. (eds). *Lectures on violence, perversion and delinquency: the Portman papers*. London, Karnac

Friedlander, K. (1947) *The psychoanalytic approach to juvenile delinquency*. London, Routledge.

Friedman, M., Glasser, M., Laufer, E., Laufer, M. & Wohl, M. (1972) Attempted suicide and self-mutilation in adolescence: some observations from a psychoanalytic research project. *The International Journal of Psychoanalysis*. 53, 179–183.

Freud, S. (1905) Infantile sexuality. Part II: Three essays on the theory of sexuality. S. E. 7

Freud, A. (1949) Aggression in relation to emotional development: normal and pathological. In: *The writings of Anna Freud*, Vol. 4. New York, International Universities Press, 1968. pp. 497–489.

Freud, A. (1965) Normality and pathology in childhood. In: *Assessments of development*. London, Hogarth Press.

Glasser, M. (1986) Identification and its vicissitudes as observed in the perversions. *The International Journal of Psychoanalysis*. 67, 9–16.

Glasser, M. (1992) Problems in the psychoanalysis of certain narcissistic disorders. *The International Journal of Psychoanalysis*. 73, 493–503.

Glasser, M. (1996) Aggression and sadism in the perversion. In: Rosen, I. (ed.) *Sexual deviation*. 3rd ed. Oxford, OUP.

Glasser, M. (1998) On violence: a preliminary communication. *The International Journal of Psychoanalysis*. 79, 887–902.

Glover, E. (1956) *The early development of the mind*. London, Imago Publishing Co., Ltd.

Glover, E. (1960) *The roots of crime*. London, International Universities Press Inc.

Goldsmith, L. (2000) Mollie Mackenzie obituary. *The Guardian* 9 May 2000.

Horne, A. (1999a) Sexual abuse and sexual abusing in childhood and adolescence. In: Lanyado, M. & Horne, A. (eds.) *The handbook of child & adolescent psychotherapy: psychoanalytic approaches*. London, Routledge.

Horne, A. (1999b) Thinking about gender in theory and practice with children and adolescents. *Journal of the British Association of Psychotherapists*. 37, 35–49.

Horne, A. (2001) Brief communications from the edge: psychotherapy with challenging adolescents. *Journal of Child Psychotherapy*. 27(1). Also, in Lanyado, M. & Horne, A. (eds.) *A question of technique*. London, Routledge, 2006. 128–142.

Horne, A. (2003) Oedipal aspirations and phallic fears: on fetishism in childhood and young adulthood. *Journal of Child Psychotherapy*. 29 (1), 37–52.

Horne, A. (2004) Gonnae no' dae that! The internal and external worlds of the delinquent adolescent. *Journal of Child Psychotherapy*. 30 (3), 330–346.

Horne, A. (2009) From intimacy to acting-out: assessment and consultation about dangerousness. In: Horne, A. & Lanyado, M. (eds.) *Through assessment to consultation: Independent psychoanalytic approaches with children and adolescents.* London, Routledge.

Horne, A. (2010) Rhythm, blues, affirmation and enactment: it's tough soloing without a rhythm section. *British Journal of Psychotherapy.* 26 (1), 1–21.

Horne, A. (2012a) Body and soul: developmental urgency and impasse. In: Horne, A. & Lanyado, M. (eds.) *Winnicott's children: Independent psychoanalytic approaches with children and adolescents.* London, Routledge.

Horne, A. (2012b) Entertaining the body in mind: thoughts on incest, the body, sexuality and the self. In: Williams, P., Keene, J. & Dermen, S. (eds.) *Independent psychoanalysis today.* London, Karnac.

Horne, A. (2012c) On delinquency. In: Horne, A. & Lanyado, M. (eds.) *Winnicott's children: Independent psychoanalytic approaches with children and adolescents* London, Routledge.

Horne, A. (2012d) Winnicott's delinquent. In: Reeves, C. (ed.) *Broken bounds: contemporary reflections on the anti-social tendency Winnicott Studies Monograph Series.* London, Karnac.

Horne, A. (2018) *On children who privilege the body: reflections of an Independent psychotherapist.* Hove & New York, Routledge.

Horne, A. (2019) Reflections on the ego ideal in childhood. In: Harding, C. (ed.) *The superego according to psycho-analysis: theoretical and clinical perspectives.* Hove & New York, Routledge.

Hurry, A. (1998) Psychoanalysis and developmental therapy. In: Hurry A. (ed.) *Psychoanalysis and developmental therapy.* London, Karnac. pp. 32–73.

Laufer, M. & Laufer, M. E. (eds.) (1989) *Developmental breakdown and psychoanalytic treatment in adolescence: clinical studies.* New Haven and London, Yale University Press.

Morgan, D. & Ruszczynski, S. (2007) The Portman clinic – an historical sketch. In: Fishman, C. & Ruszczynski, R. (eds.) *Letures on violence, perversion and delinquency: the Portman papers.* London, Karnac.

Nolleke, B. (2019) Marjorie Franklin. *Psychoanalysts. Biographical dictionary.* Available from: www.psychoanalytikerinnen.de/

Parsons, M. (2006/7) From biting teeth to biting wit: the normative development of aggression. In: Morgan, D. & Ruszczynski, S. (eds.) *Lectures on violence, perversion and delinquency: the portman papers, 2007.* London, Karnac Books. Also, in: Harding, C. (ed.) (2006) Aggression and sexuality. London, Brunner-Routledge.

Parsons, M. (2009) The roots of violence: theory and implications for technique with children and adolescents. In: Lanyado, M. & Horne, A. (eds.) *The handbook of child and adolescent psychotherapy.* Revised edition. London, Routledge.

Parsons, M. (2011) Aggression and violence in adolescents. In: Williams, P. (ed.) *Aggression: from fantasy to action.* London, Karnac.

Parsons, M. & Dermen, S. (1999) The violent child and adolescent. In: Lanyado, M. & Horne, A. (eds.) *The handbook of child and adolescent psychotherapy.* London, Routledge.

Parsons, M. & Horne, A. (2009) Anxiety, projection and the quest for magical fixes: when one is asked to assess risk. In: Horne, A. & Lanyado, M. (eds.) *Through assessment to consultation: Independent psychoanalytic approaches with children and adolescents.* London, Routledge.

Parsons, M., with Radford, P. & Horne, A. (1999) Non-intensive psychotherapy and the assessment process. In: Lanyado, M. & Horne, A. (eds.) *The handbook of child and adolescent psychotherapy.* London, Routledge.

Rodway, S. (1999) Josephine Lomax Simpson. *Obituary. The Guardian.* 12 June 1999.

Sternberg, J. (2007) A child psychotherapist's assessment tools. In: Thorpe, C. & Trowell, J. (eds.) Re–rooted lives: inter-disciplinary work within the family justice system. Bristol, Jordans.

Thomson, M. (2011) *The solution to his own enigma: connecting the life of Montague David Eder (1865–1936), socialist, psychoanalyst, zionist and modern saint. Cambridge Journal of Medical History.* 2011 Jan. 55 (1), 61–84.

Tyson, P. & Tyson, R. (1990) *Psychoanalytic theories of development: an integration.* New Haven and London, Yale University Press.

Woods, J. (2003) Boys who have abused: psychoanalytic psychotherapy with victims/perpetrators of sexual abuse. London and New York, Jessica Kingsley.

Woods, J. (2014) Seeing and being seen; the compulsive use of internet pornography through the lens of Winnicott`s thinking. In: Spelman, M. B. & Thomson-Salo, F. (eds.) *The Winnicott tradition,* London, Karnac.

Woods, J. (2016) The making of an abuser. *Journal of Child Psychotherapy.* 42 (3), 318–327.

Index

sexual abuse 48, 53, 55, 60, 86, 108, 144
sexual aggression xx, xx, 56
sexual arousal 39, 42, 54, 94
sexual enactments 138–52
sexual fantasies 22, 48–9, 56
sexualization 2, 39, 45–7, 69, 117, 119, 120, 139, 142
sexual perversion 1, 3, 141
sexual reproduction 23
sexual sadism 86–7
sexual touching 64
sexual violence 54, 86, 125
Shiva, A. 86
Shoham, S. G. 140–1
Siskind, D. 97
social media xv
social selves 67
Stern, D. 16
Stoller, R. xiv, 109
Strachey, J. 16
symbolic equation 45
Symington, N. 14–5, 19, 21

Target, M. 41
Thinking Heart, The (Alvarez) 12
Three Essays on the Theory of Sexuality (Freud) 22–3
traumas 54, 56, 69; aggressive patients witnessed 81; anxieties from 32; children act 13; children suffering 81; early stages of psychotherapy with 123–36; emotional 48, 53; impact of 159; of inadequacy 86; of long-term hospitalizations 88; perverse behaviour xx; psychopathy and 85;

referrals of patients xiii; relational x, xii; relationships in childhood 109, 144; sense of active control xii; tolerate frustration by 81; victims/perpetrators xv
Turner, J. 120
Tyson, B. 156
Tyson, P. 156

UK Council for Child Internet Safety 61

verbal abuse 40
Viding, E. 85
violence 79–90, 125, 162–3; abuse 54; addictive 10; aggression 4; in children 79–90; defined xiv; domestic 82; illustrations of 23; physical 3, 6, 11; pornography 125; predatory 25; sadistic xiv, xiv, 73; self-preservative xiv; sexual 54, 86, 125
Violence Research Workshop 157–8
voyeuristic backroom 68–9

Wales 36
Washington 23
Watts District of Los Angeles 9
Welldon, E. 108–9, 118
White, S. F. 10
Williams, H. 13
Winnicott, D. W. 15, 44, 52, 56–7, 60–2, 70, 81, 96–7, 119, 123
Wood, H. 56, 139
World Trade Centre 23
Wright, K. 59
Wuthering Heights (Bronte) 14

For Product Safety Concerns and Information please contact our EU
representative GPSR@taylorandfrancis.com
Taylor & Francis Verlag GmbH, Kaufingerstraße 24, 80331 München, Germany

9 780367 415570